KEEP SLIM AND FIT

Sally Ann Voak

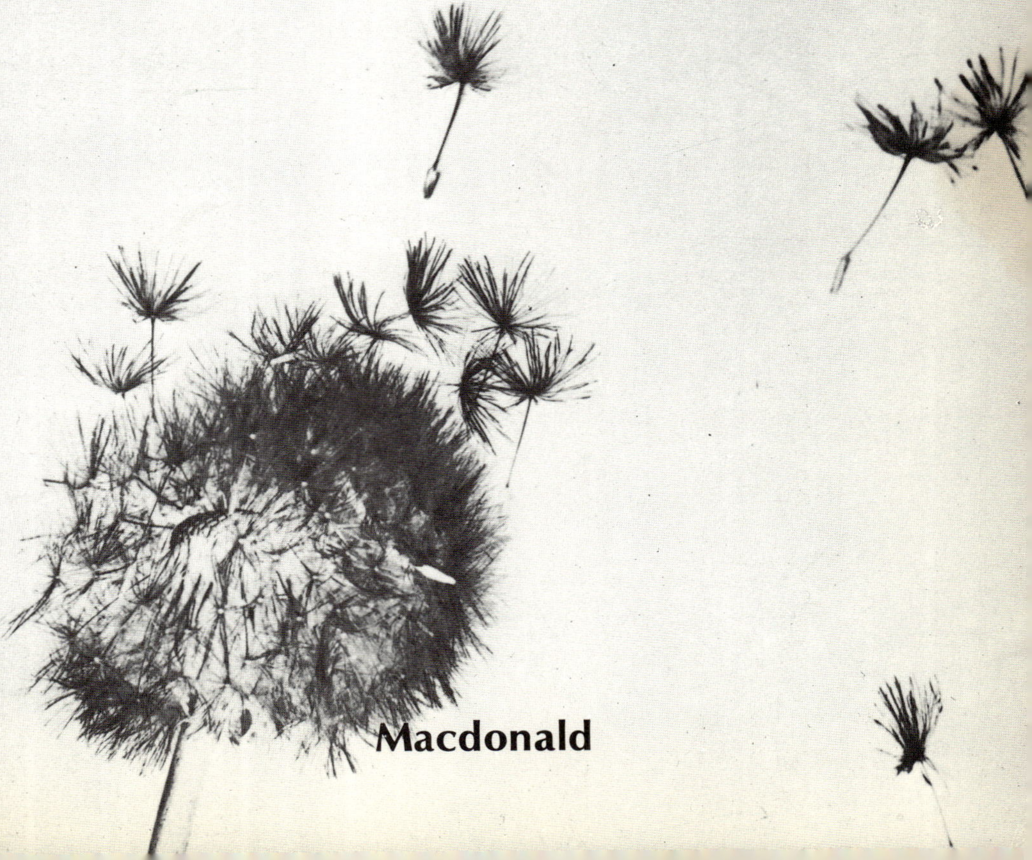

Macdonald

Editorial manager
Chester Fisher
Series editor
Jim Miles
Editor
Linda Sonntag
Designer
Michael Bilsland
Production
Penny Kitchenham

Published in association with
Thames Television's programme
After Noon Plus, edited by
Catherine Freeman

First published 1979
Macdonald Educational Ltd
Holywell House
Worship Street
London EC2A 2EN

ISBN 0 356 06206 6 (paperback edition)
ISBN 0 356 06286 4 (cased edition)

Made and printed by Waterlows
(Dunstable) Ltd

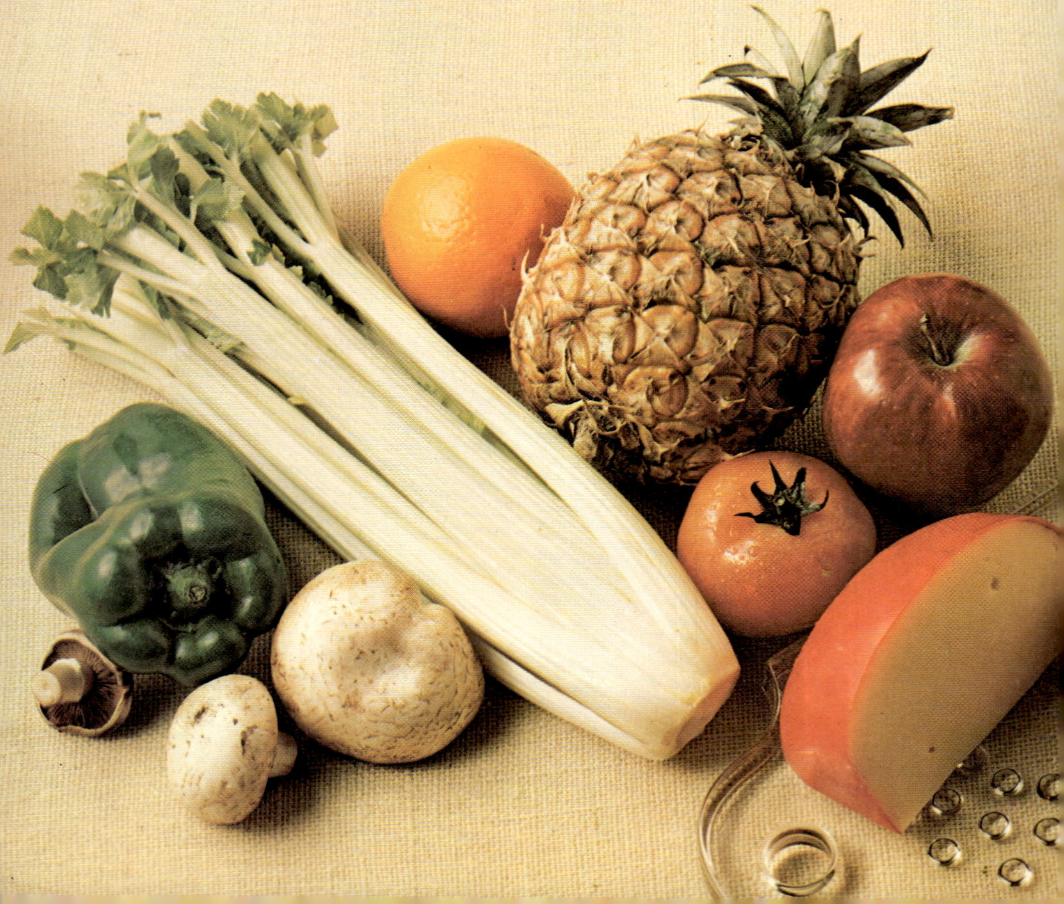

Contents

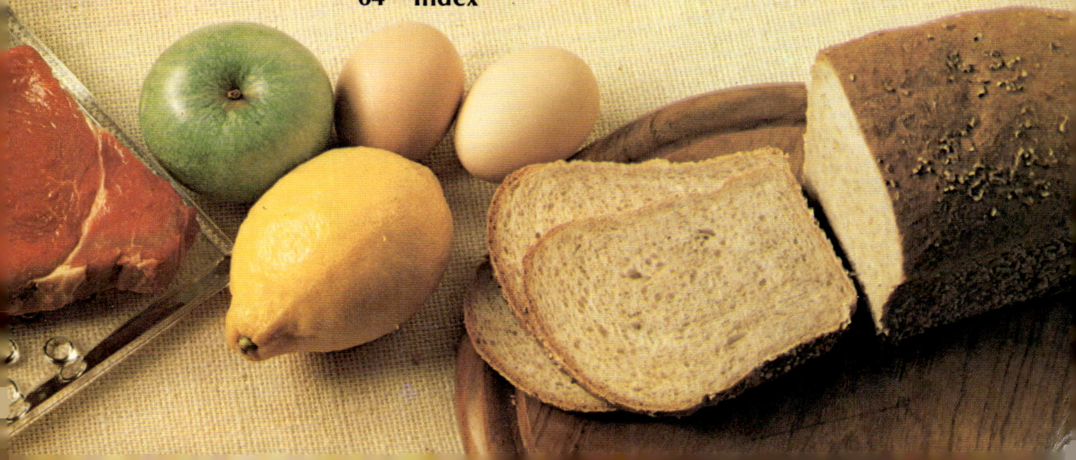

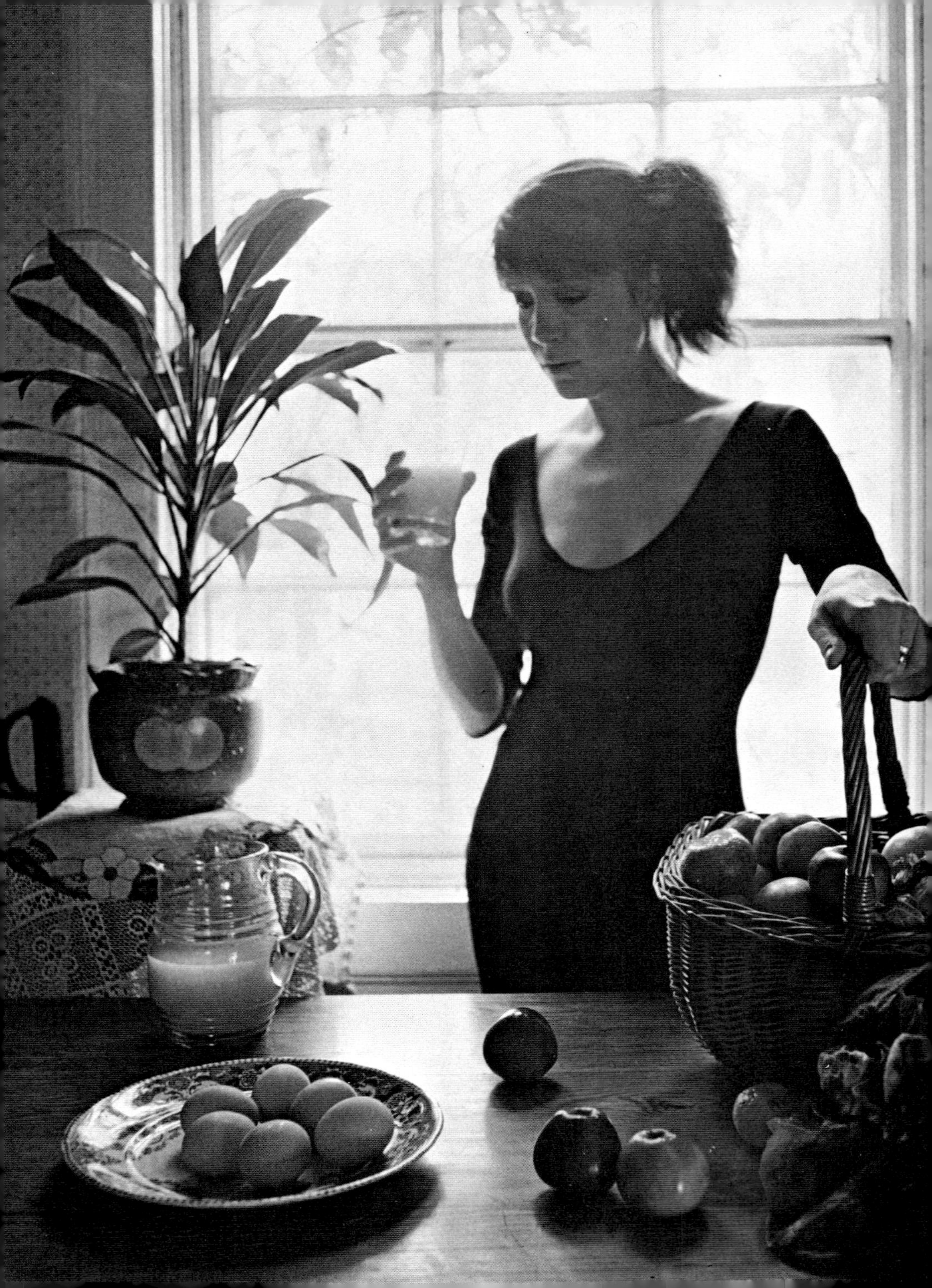

Introduction

Everyone wants to be slim, and most people have tried to lose weight, successfully or unsuccessfully, at one time or another. Spring and summer are the favourite seasons for slimmers, but unfortunately, that sudden decision to shed the pounds often means going on a gimmick diet and failing to follow it up with a sensible long-term eating plan.

Panic measures usually give only short-term results. The pounds soon pile on again and you're back to square one. There really is no magic way to lose weight and stay fit. Keeping in trim must be part of life itself. If it's enjoyable you'll stick with it and your slimming campaign is likely to be successful.

This book aims to provide you with incentive, encouragement and bright ideas on all aspects of staying trim. We believe that it is possible to combine slimming with delicious gourmet eating, and even drinking. This book contains 13 different diets and over 30 delicious Calorie-counted recipes. Naturally the dishes are simple to cook too and are geared around particular needs: from couples who love to entertain to slimming children and even babies.

Fitness can also be fun as well as good for you. That's why our exercise plan has been specially devised to start with very gentle movements and work progressively up to more strenuous ones as you become gradually fitter.

There's also an informative section packed with the latest facts and findings on nutrition and human metabolism, and a comprehensive Calorie chart to help you plan your own menus.

So if you feel overweight and below par, don't panic. Try the diets and exercises in this book and you *will* get slim. You'll have *fun* too.

Slimming and your health

A healthy body is a slim body: of that doctors are agreed. But luckily it's no longer fashionable to be painfully thin; the 17-inch waistline of the 18th and 19th centuries, the tiny hips of the 20s and the skinny legs of the swinging 60s have been superseded by a slightly more curvy look. A look which is slim, but not thin. The illustration below shows how fashion has dictated the shape of the female body through the ages. Today, fashion is health: swinging shiny hair, clear skin and bright eyes.

Since fashion is now so sensible, why is it that half the people in this country are overweight? The medical evidence that overweight is unhealthy is now overwhelming. Most doctors consider that obesity is a disease; a disease that will shorten your expected lifespan dramatically (Metropolitan Life Insurance Company figures show that if you're 20 per cent overweight your expected lifespan is shortened by 25 per cent). If you're fat you are more likely to suffer from digestive and respiratory complaints, backache, diabetes and heart disease. So why are so many of us 20 per cent – or more – over the top? And why do doctors repeatedly report failure in treating obese patients? For the sad fact is that the majority of slimmers put weight back on as quickly as they take it off.

The answer to the first question is that modern society is food-and-drink orientated to the point of the ridiculous. From the very first time a mother offers her baby a soggy rusk to stop a tantrum, food becomes much more than a means of satisfying hunger; it becomes a love-offering, a weapon, a comfort.

The answer to the second question is that most dieters see their slimming as a short-term campaign to lose a specific

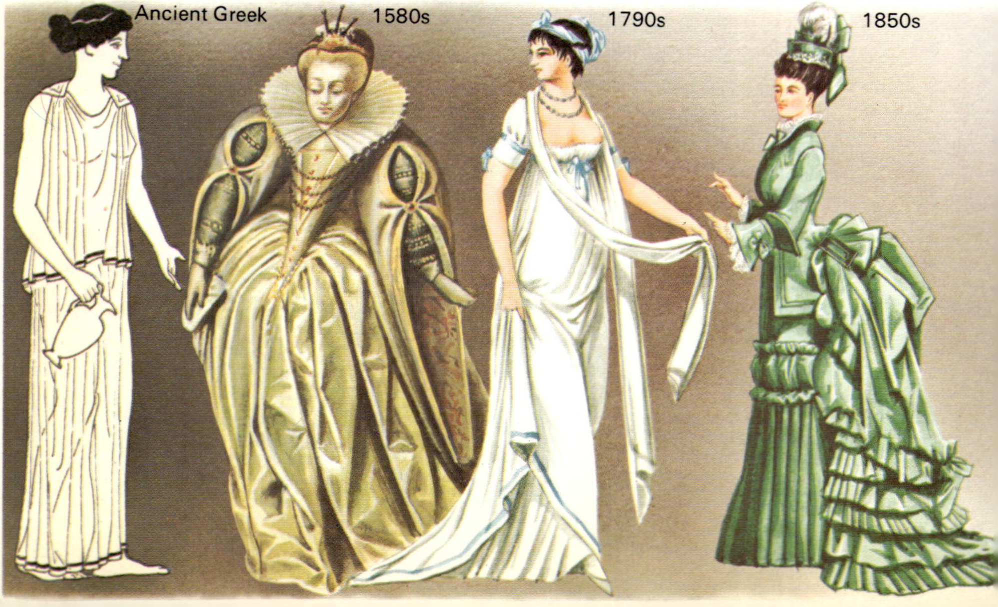

amount of weight; once that weight-loss has been achieved, then the only thing to do is to put it back on again: they don't understand that achieving a healthy, slim body must be a lifelong aim with a positive approach to good eating, linked to a sensible exercise programme. Obviously most of us will have the occasional relapse, where weight tends to pile on, but the healthy sensible thing is not to let the situation get out of hand but to tackle the problem immediately.

Are you overweight? Charts giving the 'ideal' weight ranges according to height and bone structure are readily available, but these can be misleading. Nowadays doctors use skinfold thickness calipers to measure a fold of flesh at various points of the body (your GP, slimming club doctor or nutritionist will do this for you) and you can use your thumb and forefinger for a similar test. Simply pinch the back of your upper arm, or your midriff or tummy; if you can pinch a thickness of more than an inch you're probably too fat. Your mirror is also a reliable visual guide to overweight. Strip off (if you have the courage) and look at your reflection. Don't kid yourself if you are clearly bulging all over the place. Scales are the most obvious weight-checking guide; use the same ones, at the same time of day and position your feet evenly. Don't forget that fluid fluctuations (just before your period, for instance) can sometimes give a misleading reading.

If you weighed less than you do now when you were younger, then you are also probably overweight. There's a common misconception that the middle-aged *should* put on a few pounds, or stones for 'health'. This is untrue. Older people need less energy from food in the form of Calories as they take less exercise, but their weight should remain the same.

If you feel breathless, below par and find shirt-buttons keep popping then you could also lose a few kilos, even if your contemporaries are equally solidly built and don't seem to be worrying about it.

Are you ready to improve your shape, *and* your health? If you have the inclination, now is the time to check with your doctor. The chances are that he will encourage you to start right away.

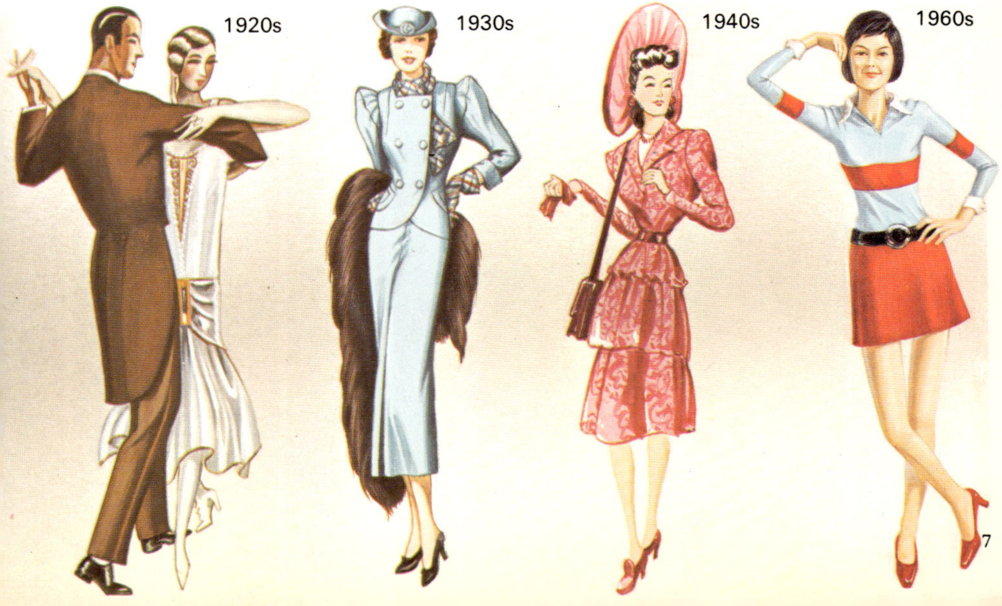

Food that figures

For slimmers, there is no magic combination of foods which can strip away excess weight: what's needed is a balanced selection of foods which provide the maximum nutritional value for the low number of Calories needed to regulate weight. Your daily foods should come from these groups:

Proteins (meat, fish, cheese, eggs, milk, cereals, nuts) are the essential constituents of the millions of microscopic cells which make up the blood, tissues and organs. They are vital for growth, repair and maintenance. Protein foods supply about 112 Calories per 25g (1oz) and have the advantage of giving sustained energy over quite a long period of time.

Carbohydrates (sugar, starchy foods, confectionary, pastries, bread, puddings) provide energy and about the same number of Calories as protein foods. However, they often do little else besides, and so they frequently need to be limited on a slimming diet. The exception is bread, which supplies vitamins and minerals as well as energy. Carbohydrate foods also have the disadvantage of giving an instant energy boost which is followed by a lowering of blood sugar, resulting in a feeling of hunger.

Fats provide a concentrated source of energy, make food more palatable and help you feel satisfied. They are high in Calories (100g (4oz) butter, which is mostly fat, provides 800 Calories), but several of the important vitamins, particularly A, D and E are found dissolved in fat in foods like butter, milk and margarine. You will certainly get all the nutrients you need from fat if you include a certain amount of milk, cheese and egg yolk in your diet.

Vitamins are essential for health because they enable the body to make use of other nutrients. Until this century they were unknown, but now research is revealing much more about their function, and new

Fried bread with bacon, porridge with milk and sugar and tea: 1000 Calories, no vitamin C and plenty of fat!

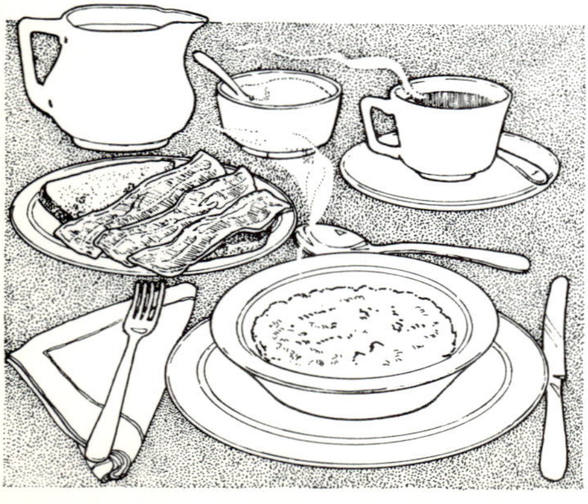

Orange juice, boiled egg, crispbreads and low-fat spread, unsweetened tea: 350 Calories, protein, vitamin C and some carbohydrate.

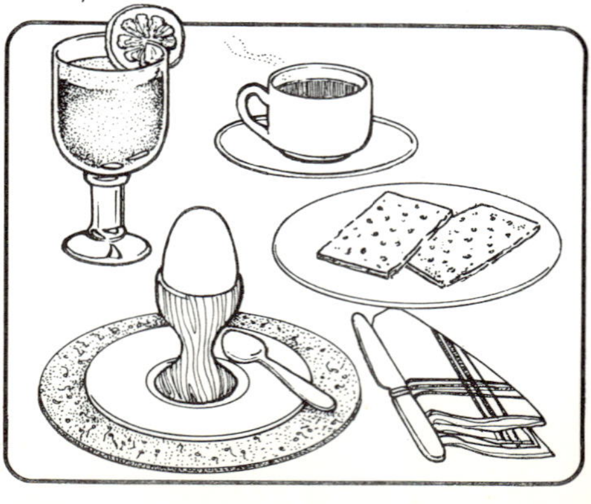

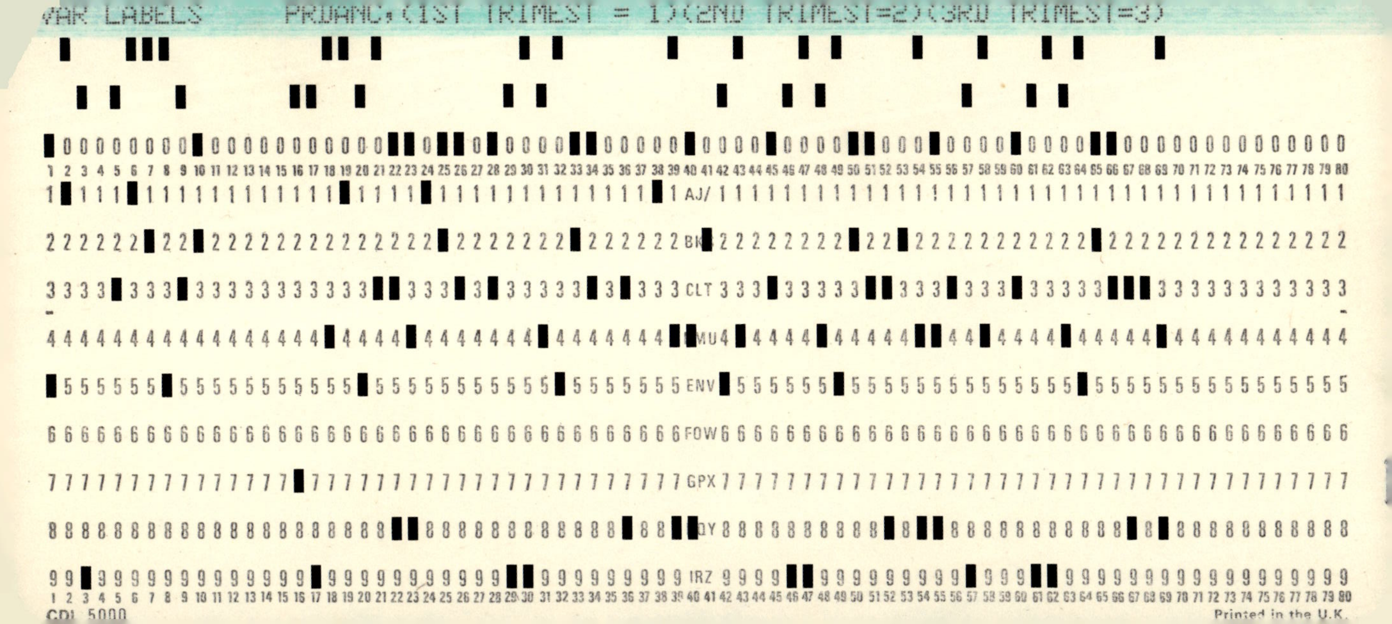
VAR LABELS PRVANC,(1ST TRIMEST = 1)(2ND TRIMEST=2)(3RD TRIMEST=3)
CDI 5000
Printed in the U.K.

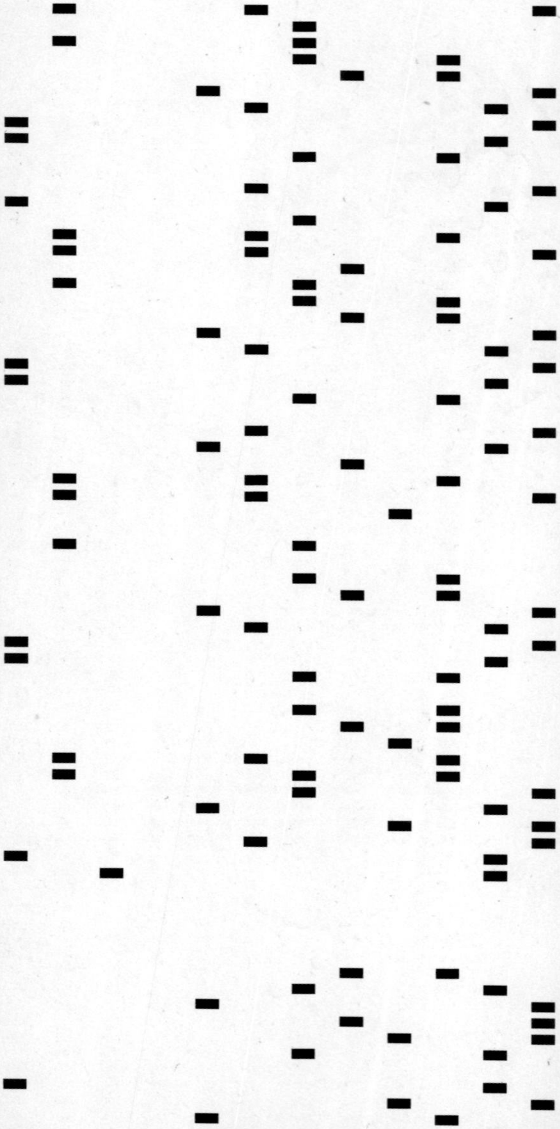

vitamin functions are being discovered.
Vitamin A (fish liver oils, animal liver, eggs, milk, butter, carrots) is essential for body growth, eye function, resistance to infection.
Vitamin B1 (thiamine) (wheatgerm, yeast, wholemeal bread, lean meat) is essential for carbohydrate metabolism, nerves, digestion, the heart.
Vitamin B2 (riboflavin) (yeast, wheatgerm, liver, kidney, cheese, meat) is for skin, nails, hair. A deficiency leads to dull hair, split fingernails, itchy eyes.
Vitamin B6 (pyridoxine) (wheatgerm, yeast, liver, potatoes) is vital for healthy skin, proper growth in children.
Nicotinic acid (yeast, wheat, bread, liver, meat, fish) is for healthy skin, mucous membranes and the nervous system.
Pantothenic acid (yeast, liver, beans) helps burn up fat for energy and is essential for fluid balance.
Folic acid (yeast, liver, milk, green vegetables) and *Vitamin B12 (cynacocoblamin)* (liver, meat, wholemeal bread, wheatgerm) are both essential for healthy blood.
Vitamin C (ascorbic acid) (oranges, lemon, grapefruit) is for vitality, resistance to infection, and strengthens the connective tissues which make healthy bones, teeth, blood, vessels.
Vitamin D (calciferol) (fish liver oils, eggs, milk, sunshine) regulates the calcium and phosphorous content of the body and is essential for the bone formation of children and embryos.
Vitamin E (tocopherol) (wheatgerm, whole grains, wholewheat bread, nuts, vegetable oils) protects body tissues and keeps blood circulating freely.
Vitamin K (green vegetables, tomatoes, liver, carrot tops, soya bean oil) is essential to prevent blood clotting.
Minerals are also essential for health. Calcium is the best known (in milk, cheese) and is essential for the formation of bones, teeth, hair, fingernails and all body cells. Iron (in egg yolk, liver) helps make blood and deficiency causes anaemia. It's vital for women during the child-bearing years and *must* be included in your slimming diet.
Dietary fibre is not a nutrient but it is the roughage which assists digestion and the passage of food through the body. Current medical opinion suggests that dietary fibre is more vital for healthy living than was previously thought. (More about this subject on p. 28).

Hamburger, chips and peas, fizzy drink and cake: more than 1,500 Calories and very little protein.

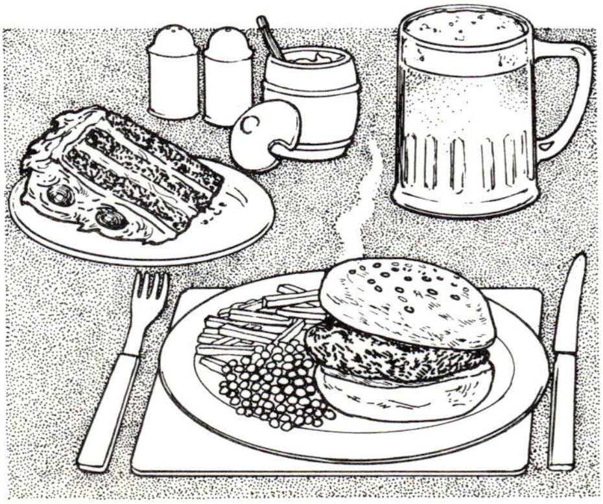

Chicken salad, mineral water and an apple: about 350 Calories plus vitamins, minerals and protein.

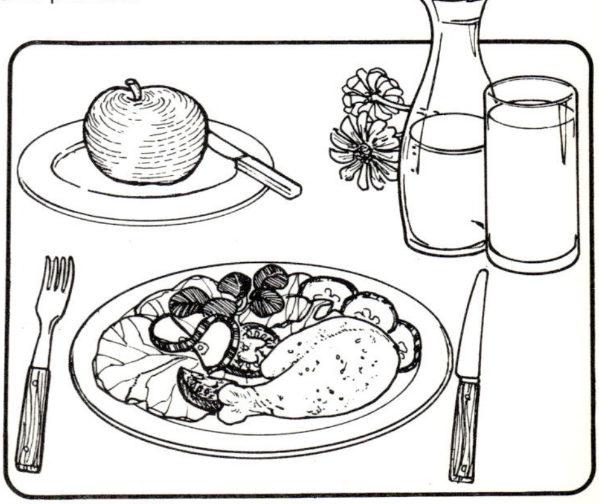

Calories and your lifestyle

If you have followed slimming diets before, you will be familiar with the unit of energy measurement called the Calorie. This is the amount of heat needed to raise the temperature of one kilogram of water by one degree centigrade and it should, to be accurate, be referred to as the kiloCalorie. If you get a diet sheet from your doctor or hospital it is quite likely to be calculated in kiloCalories. However, a new measurement, the kiloJoule (kJ) is being introduced which may, eventually, replace the Calorie. Since one Calorie is the equivalent of 4.184 kJ, the new measurement does give rather unwieldy figures to play with, so in this book we shall be referring to Calories with the kiloJoule equivalent given in the diet and recipe section only.

Calories and energy

How much energy do we need each day, and how can we step up our rate of energy expenditure? The energy requirements vary according to the individual, not just in the kind of job he does and lifestyle he leads but in the way his body uses energy in processes like heartbeat, breathing and the chemical reactions between cells.

1.4 Calories per minute

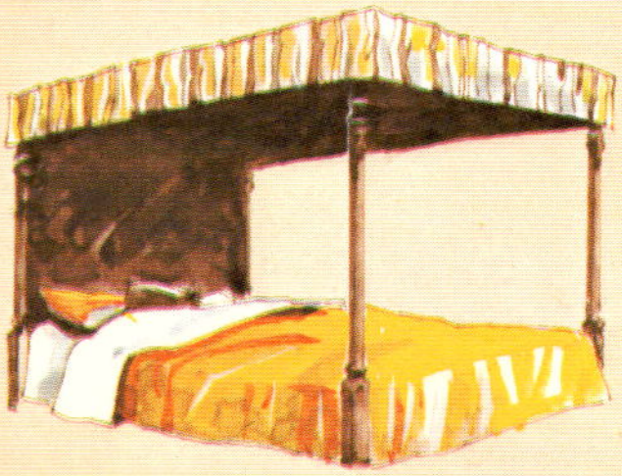

Because the energy output is such a finely balanced, individual thing, charts and figures can only provide a rough guide to the needs of each person. But we do know that when the energy intake is less than the energy output, the body will draw on fat reserves for fuel and *you will lose weight.*

Metabolism

Even if you do nothing at all during the day, your bodily processes continue and you burn Calories. This is known as the basal metabolic rate and is more or less proportional to the surface area of your skin. It changes with age, increasing until the age of about 25, decreasing after 35. Unfairly women have a lower basal metabolic rate than men. On average, men require about 2700-3000 Calories a day, while women need only about 2200-2500 (and some of us would grow plump on even that amount!).

2.5–4.9 Calories per minute

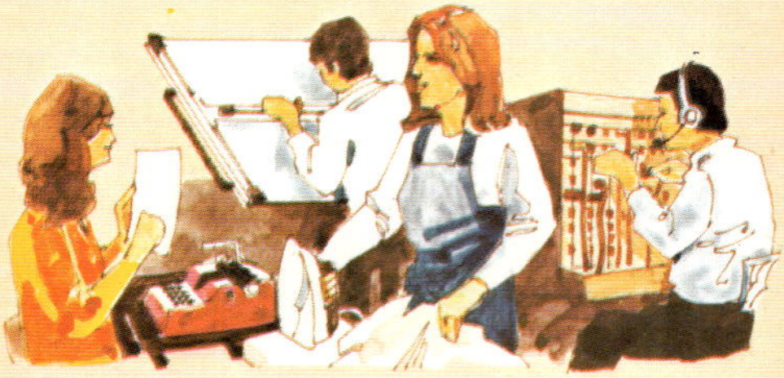

This illustration shows how many Calories you need to keep you going in your sort of work.

Who needs what

The illustration on this page gives an idea of how the Calories are burnt up during various activities. You can speed up your bodily fuel-burning process effectively by walking, taking regular exercise, dancing, and enjoying sport. If you calculated the weight lost per 1000 Calories burned you would be disappointed, but there is evidence that exercise affects a more lasting, more efficient fat-burning process that carries on after the exercise is finished. However, to be effective, exercise should always be regular.

Carbohydrates

Carbohydrates, measured in units of 5g, are also used in slimming diets. The two methods are often confused. Basically, carbohydrate-unit counting is simply another method of counting Calories. Foods that are rich in carbohydrates (sugar, biscuits, sweets and cakes) provide plenty of Calories of energy and usually not much else. So, by cutting down drastically on carbohydrate intake (which accounts for about half your normal daily Calorie intake) and *not* increasing your protein and fat intake you should automatically substantially reduce Calories without upsetting the nutritional value of the diet. The catch in this slimming method comes with alcohol which, although low in carbohydrate, is high in Calories. A good low-carbohydrate diet takes this into account by restricting alcohol.

In this book, we have used Calories for diet calculations, but we do give a guide to the carbohydrate value (in units of 5g) in the charts which begin on p. 60.

5.0–7.4 Calories per minute

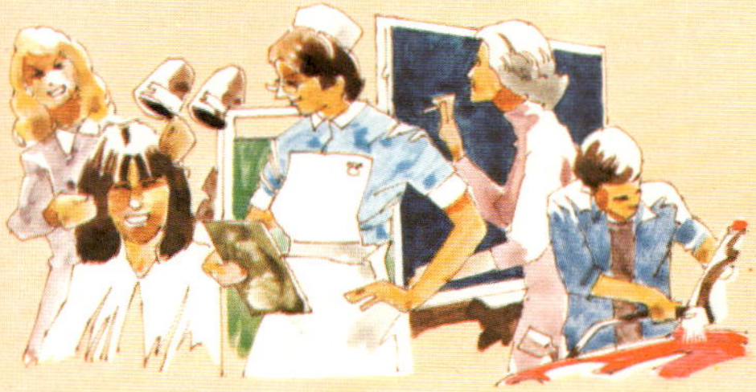

7.5–9.0 Calories per minute

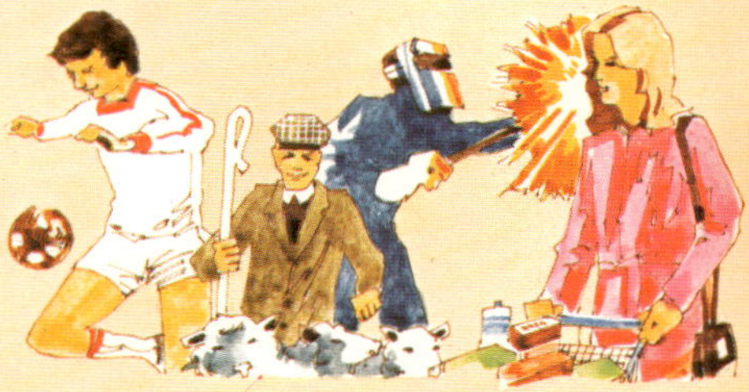

50 Calorie fruit portions

1 large fresh apple
4 fresh apricots
1 small banana
Just under 227g (9oz) fresh blackberries
About 20 fresh eating cherries
Just under 227g (9oz) fresh blackcurrants or redcurrants
130g (5oz) fresh damsons
2-3 fresh figs
About 130g (5oz) fresh gooseberries
18-20 fresh black grapes
About 15 fresh green grapes
2 large fresh grapefruits
750ml (1¼ pints) fresh lemon juice
227g (9oz) fresh loganberries
1 300g (10oz) Canteloupe melon
1 large nectarine
1 large fresh orange
150ml (¾ pint) fresh orange juice
1 large fresh peach
1½ fresh pears
2 thin slices fresh pineapple
2 large fresh plums
3 small prunes
175g (6oz) fresh raspberries
1225g (3lb) fresh rhubarb

Metabolism and slimming

It is now accepted that the metabolism (or the rate at which the body uses energy in processes like heartbeat, breathing and chemical reactions between cells) of a fat or potentially fat person is quite different from that of a slim person. A fat person 'ticks over' more slowly than a slim one and is predisposed to store fat more efficiently. Although this trait can start right from childhood, changes in circumstances and lifestyle can slow you down. For instance, a woman who has spent five years having babies has had her whole body geared to storing fat during that time and she probably has to re-adjust to a slower life than she was used to as a working girl. The man who has switched from an unsettled bachelor existence to a settled family life is also probably eating more and exercising less.

Exercise is a good way to rev up a sluggish metabolism; it is now believed that regular exercise encourages the fat-burning processes for quite a while after the exercise stops. Also, taking smaller meals more regularly can make your bodily processes shift into top gear again: you'll lose weight at a faster rate than if you consumed the same amount of Calories in two large meals during the day and you'll feel livelier too.

Drugs

What about drugs? Amphetamines were devised to cure a condition in which people would suddenly fall asleep in the middle of normal activities like talking or driving, but later it was found that they also curbed appetite by working on the appetite-controlling centres in the brain. Unfortunately, these drugs were discovered to be addictive. There are similar, but safer, drugs available to help slimmers but these are usually only prescribed in really tough cases under hospital supervision. There is one school of thought that obesity, as a dangerous disease, should in certain cases be treated with continuous drug therapy, but unfortunately most slimmers do put weight back on as soon as drug therapy ceases. However, for most dieters it is best to endeavour to lose weight without the help of drugs. Let your willpower do the work with the help of a sensible diet.

Do you use food as a tranquillizer? Some American researchers have found that certain fatties (usually women) actually slow down their own metabolism by reaching for food at times of stress. This has a doubly bad effect: the extra food puts on extra weight that is increased by the slower metabolic rate. As soon as the victim tries to slim, she will become twitchy and complain that life is too complicated. The answer here is that a little stress is *good* for you, especially if it gets your body working. If you know that this is your problem, it makes sense to prepare for a few nervy moments by channelling the extra energy into something useful such as a decorating project or your work. Don't leave yourself time to worry about being worried.

Are you on the Pill? If you are, then your body is on a continuous 'phantom pregnancy' and is probably going to store fat on breasts, tummy and hips. You may find that you need to cut your daily Calorie intake by as much as 10 per cent to stay slim. If you have a nagging weight problem and/or other symptoms such as fluid retention and leg cramps it's advisable to see your doctor immediately. The 'mini' Pills such as Femulen, Micronor, Neogest, Noriday and Microval are low in oestrogen and produce fewer side-effects, including fewer weight problems. (Don't forget that any pill containing oestrogen, whether prescribed as a contraceptive, for your skin, or to regulate periods may cause weight gain.)

A change of lifestyle

Have you had an operation? Your metabolism may slow down following a hysterectomy of gall bladder operation or other surgery and you may also be forced to cut down on exercise which will contribute to your weight problems. The best way to play it is to get moving again as soon as your doctor allows you to, and to avoid overeating immediately after surgery and during convalescence. Well-meaning relatives may encourage you to eat too much: go for a high-protein diet with iron-rich foods and green vegetables and cut out those chocolates and sweets. See your doctor, too, about taking vitamin supplements.

Have you retired? It isn't just the extra food and lack of exercise that makes men, particularly, put on weight after retirement, it's the sudden feeling of relaxation after a lifetime of responsibilities, plus the natural slowing down of metabolism that occurs in the later years. To stay slim, you *must* cut Calories and step up regular, gentle exercise such as walking. For women, retirement doesn't bring the same degree of relaxation but the menopause can be accompanied by weight problems. Some doctors believe that the function of weight-gain in the menopause is the enlargement of existing fat cells and that it is advisable to decrease your Calorie intake by five percent every five years after the age of 40.

Fat and feminism

There is no doubt that women have a tougher time losing weight than men. Our hormones, metabolism and domestic responsibilities seem to conspire against us losing weight. Men are not prone to fluctuations in fluid or (obviously) the problems of pregnancy and lactation, and they can lose weight almost twice as fast as women. What's more they can keep weight off more successfully than women. are able to.

Feminists go even further than that: they maintain that women use fat as a response to sexual inequality, as protection, as a means of assertion, as a weapon. It can help to take a leaf from the feminists' book and stand back from the Calorie-counting for a while to examine your feelings about yourself and your role in life. Self-help groups with discussion on topics such as the differences between fat and thin, what it really means to *you* to be fat, and just what place food has in your life, can be very successful. At home, you can make a list of what you eat and try to remember *why* you ate it, and what you felt at the time.

Psychology and slimming

Doctors and slimming experts are finding that the combination of sensible dieting and a positive psychological approach to obesity can be very successful in promoting weight-loss, even in the most extreme cases. You can join a slimming club and take part in behaviour therapy and psychological counselling sessions, but it is your attitude at home that will bring you eventual success.

Think positive! Exercise a little willpower and you'll be surprised how quickly your resistance to fattening food and drink will build up. Keep thinking slim, and soon you'll match up to your ideal!

Slimming facts and fallacies

Recent research on the causes of and possible cures for obesity has revealed that some of the 'fallacies' used as excuses for fatties to go on being fatties do, in fact, have some truth in them. But there are still many misconceptions about overweight, its causes and treatment, and the issues are further confused because even the nutritionists and scientists researching the subject cannot agree on a number of points. Many interesting projects are now taking place, particularly in the field of metabolic research, but until these experiments are collated (and applied to humans as well as laboratory rats!) only vague assumptions can be drawn from them. In the meantime, here's a guide to the current thinking on those other slimming 'assumptions' we all know so well:

Fad diets The grapefruit diet, the banana and milk diet, the egg and tomato diet: we've all heard about these 'wonder' diets and the miraculous results they bring. But the truth is that there is no such thing as a 'wonder' food: grapefruit, for instance, certainly does *not* 'chew up and dissolve' body fat. Some of these diets work because they are based on the low carbohydrate principle which successfully cuts Calories because it limits the carbohydrate foods on the slimmer's menu and includes protein foods which are more satisfying, so the slimmer eats less of them. It's as simple as that. Others are based on the assumption (correct!) that a slimmer can only eat so much of one food (such as bananas) and that is probably going to total fewer Calories than the dieter's normal intake: so he will lose weight. True, but unfortunately as soon as he returns to a normal diet those pounds will pile up again. Beware of any diet that excludes all foods from one or more food group: it is bound to be detrimental to your health in the long run. An example is the protein-only diet which was popular in the United

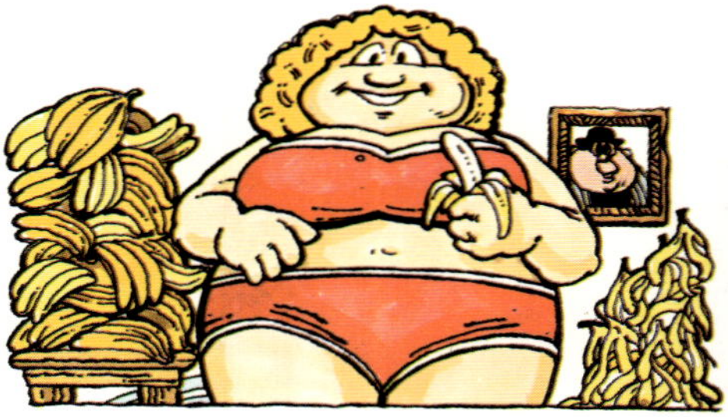

States a few years ago. This cuts carbohydrates to a dangerously low level and gave slimmers bad breath and constipation. They lost weight but also lost friends and temper!

Spot reduction Massage, faradic exercise machines and vibrator belts *won't* help you lose weight. However, they will certainly help circulation, and faradic muscular exercise machines will tone up your muscles. The problem with the latter is that the muscles soon become slack again if the machine is not used regularly. Some beauticians recommend the deep massage of the 'G5' rubber roller machine to mobilize fat tissue from specific problem areas such as bottom and hips. However, doctors do *not* agree that it is possible to choose where you want to lose weight. Another area where experts disagree is in the slimming problem called cellulite. According to continental doctors this condition, which affects hips and tummy and gives a lumpy 'orange-peel' look to the skin is caused by fluid trapped in the skin's

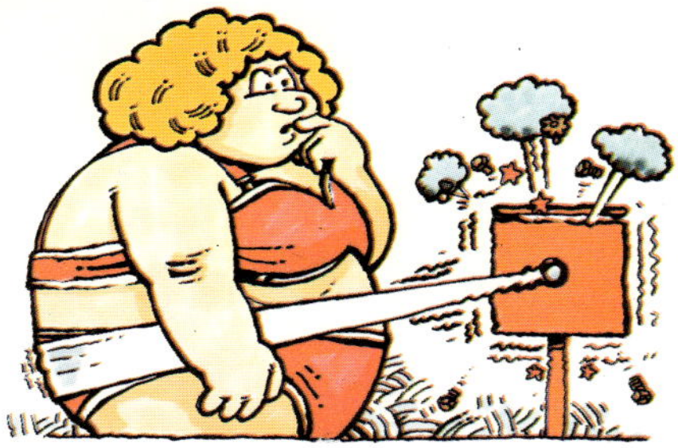

subcutaneous tissues. British doctors say it's just fat. However, treatments in the form of deep massage and a sensible diet including lots of green vegetables and salads do seem to help.

Hypnotism Some slimmers have reported 'miracle' weight-loss with the help of hypnotism. The human being is certainly extremely suggestible and becomes more so under hypnosis. If positive ideas can be implanted in the mind in this state, it can certainly help you to slim (rather like the psychological ideas of treatment described on p. 13). In the same way, cassettes and records giving psychotherapy sessions in your own home can be helpful. However, both these methods can only provide motivation; cutting those Calories is the only way to lose weight.

Fluid retention Women retain fluid just before a period which can certainly mess up their slimming efforts by giving a misleading scales reading. This can be up to 3kg (over 6lbs) if you are on the Pill. It's fine for doctors to say that the healthy body rids itself of excess water and this has

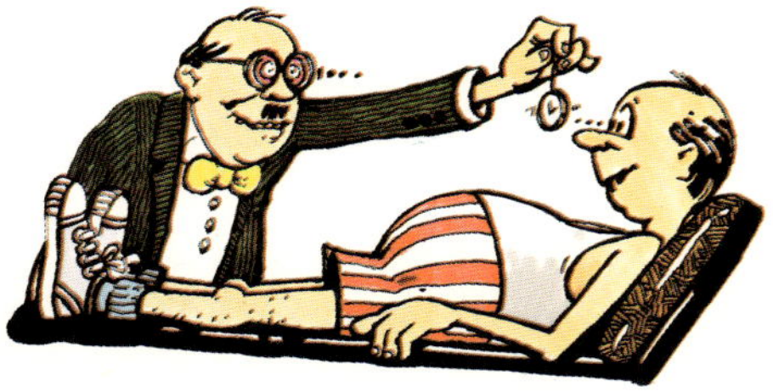

nothing to do with weight-loss, but in practice it can be very discouraging. Certain antibiotics, anti-inflammatory drugs, cortisone and oestrogen make you retain water. So do carbohydrates and salt. If you feel this could be your problem (and it often has the pre-menstrual effect of making you feel edgy as well as dumpy), then consult your doctor. Diurectic pills are available which include potassium, thus preventing potassium loss which can be a dangerous side-effect. However these should be prescribed under medical supervision. 'Water' pills and injections can lead to dehydration if used unscrupulously.

Family fatness Metabolic defects leading to overweight can be inherited. So can the behaviour patterns and eating habits associated with family fatness. In fact, if you come from a family of fatties you are very likely indeed to be fat yourself. However, while the metabolic problems are more difficult to treat, you can try to break loose from the bad eating habits of a lifetime by gradually learning to eat less, and to eat the right kind of foods. Slimming clubs and groups often report success in retraining the eating habits of whole families. It's important to make the effort, for yourself and the next generation.

Spring slimming Some slimmers claim that they can't slim in winter, but find it much easier to lose weight in spring. This phenomenon can be explained in terms of hormones. It is true that the human animal still feels a primitive need to store fat for the winter and that our mating urges rev up in the spring, reaching a peak in June and July. Many people feel comforted by eating solid, warming stews in winter, and only motivated to slim by the thought of sunny beaches and lighter, more revealing clothes. However, there are no hard and fast rules, and as soon as you feel the urge to slim, for whatever reason, you should act on it!

Choosing a good diet

You've decided you need to lose weight, so now sit down and think about the kind of diet you should follow. On the next 26 pages, you'll find a selection of diets for different people, and one will be right for you.

Dos and don'ts

Don't try to lose weight too quickly (on the Quick weight loss diet on p.20 for instance) if you are in a hectic job and know that you're short on will-power. Choose something a little more practical like the Health and beauty diet on p.18.

Do allow yourself to be inspired by the delicious-sounding dishes on the menu for your chosen diet: slimming should be fun as well as healthy.

Do be absoloutely determined to start your diet tomorrow (or even today, if that is practical). Read through the food requirements and make a special trip to the shops to stock up with the right foods. Don't forget that quite a few foods are readily interchangable. For instance, you can swap around the leafy green vegetables mentioned according to season and availability, as these have approximately the same Calorie value. When a food is unobtainable, select an alternative from the same food group with the same approximate Calorie value from the chart which starts on p 60. Never be put off a diet by one or two foods which may be unpalatable or difficult to obtain: there is always a suitable substitute.

Socializing is probably the biggest hazard in your way. If you have to go out to eat follow these rules: in a restaurant, always order clear soup as a starter. This will help to take the edge off your appetite and control it. Order plain lean meat or fish and green vegetables without potatoes or chips as your main course. Follow up with fresh fruit or fruit salad for dessert. If you go out to dinner, don't mention your diet to the hostess. Just eat a very little of everything and cut those Calories the next day. In a pub, order one short drink and keep topping it up with low-Calorie mixers. That way no-one will notice that you are not drinking the hard stuff. Of course, if you are following the Wine diet on p.22 you may drink half a bottle of dry wine daily.

Cooking for your diet and your family can be easy if you follow certain basic rules (which would be beneficial to them as well as to you). Avoid over-cooking vegetables: if they are crisp and bulky they'll seem more satisfying and will also supply more healthy fibre. Don't fry anything, even for the children. Grilling, steaming and roasting cut Calories and are far healthier too as they control the family's fat intake. Serve all meals on individual plates and not in a communal pot so that you won't be tempted to take a second helping. If there are any leftovers after a meal, *don't* eat them up yourself: you'll be doing untold damage to your Calorie count!

To make sure you stay the course, it's a good idea to keep a chart or diary of your progress. Weigh yourself once a week (not more often than that), in the early morning without clothes and on the same scales. Don't be disappointed if your weight-loss is dramatic for the first seven days and then falls off in the second and third weeks. In the first week, your weight-loss will be boosted by fluid-loss, but in the weeks to follow all you will lose is fat.

How to plan your daily eating habits

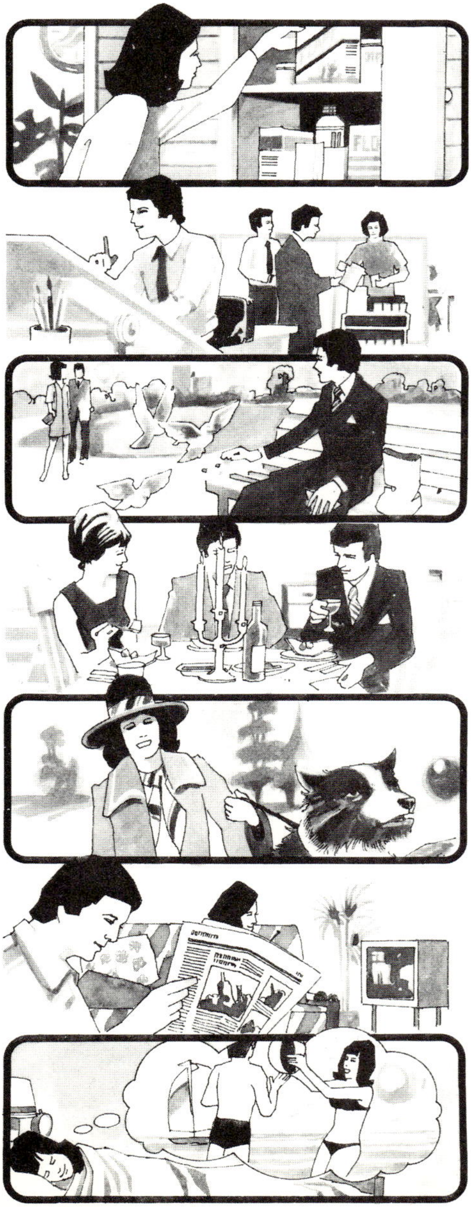

8am Before breakfast check the larder and fridge for the day's diet foods. Place all other foods out of sight in tins or at the back of the shelves. Eat your breakfast. Prepare your packed lunch.

10.30am When the coffee and snack trolley comes round, be far too busy to look at the fattening things on it. Get a colleague to fetch you an unsweetened coffee. Back to work quickly: don't watch the others eating.

1pm Take exercise at lunchtime. Eat your packed lunch in the park away from crowded cafés. Afterwards, window-shop for clothes, not food. Don't use your lunch hour to read magazines containing recipes and adverts for food.

6.30pm Make your evening meal an occasion. Set the table carefully. Eat slowly, chewing each mouthful 50 times. Enjoy good conversation but *don't* watch tv, listen to the radio or read while you eat.

8pm Take the dog for a walk around the block or go jogging after dinner. Don't settle down in front of the tv (those food ads will make you feel hungry) too early in the evening. Develop a new interest and pursue it.

10pm If you do finally succumb to the temptations of the tv, arm yourself with knitting, crochet or some work from the office to fill the gap when those hunger pangs start. Keep a bowl of raw vegetables for emergencies.

11pm Check the kitchen before you go to bed. Don't leave food around for midnight sandwich orgies. Look at holiday brochures, or read a novel in bed. Imagine the new, slim you before you finally close your eyes.

Health and beauty diet

If you're feeling jaded and are up to 7kg (1 stone) overweight, then follow the diet below for as long as you need to. You will lose weight, slowly but surely, at the rate of about 1kg (2 lbs) per week, and you will also notice that your skin begins to feel smoother, your eyes to sparkle and your hair to shine.

This diet includes all the beauty foods: protein for growth and repair of cells and tissues; vitamins A, B, C, D, E and K; minerals for healthy bones and teeth and iron for healthy blood. It also allows you 3 slices of wholewheat bread per day: don't leave this out, as it's a fund of excellent beauty nutrients and contains roughage to keep you regular.

About 1500 Calories
Daily allowance:
450ml (¾ pint) fresh, whole milk for use in tea or coffee; 3 medium slices wholewheat bread; 15g (½ oz) butter; bowl of raw vegetables for nibbling.

DAY ONE
Breakfast: ½ grapefruit (no sugar, use sweetener if you like); 1 poached egg on toast from allowance; tea or coffee with milk from allowance.
Lunch: 2 lean slices ham; large mixed salad; bread from allowance; 50 Calorie fruit portion (p.11).
Supper: Small grilled mackerel; French beans and green side-salad tossed in lemon juice; small piece cheese; bread from allowance.

DAY TWO
Breakfast: 2 lean slices bacon, grilled; 2 tomatoes, grilled; glass of orange juice (unsweetened); bread and butter from allowance; tea or coffee with milk from allowance.
Lunch: Small hamburger steak (no bun); mixed salad with lemon juice dressing; bread and butter from allowance; tea or coffee with milk from allowance; 50 Calorie fruit portion (p.11).
Supper: Soufflé omelette with citrus and avocado salad (p.51); natural yogurt with nuts, wheatgerm and chopped apple stirred in; bread and butter from allowance; tea or coffee.

DAY THREE
Breakfast: Grapefruit juice (small glass); small grilled or poached kipper; bread and butter from allowance; tea or coffee with milk from allowance.

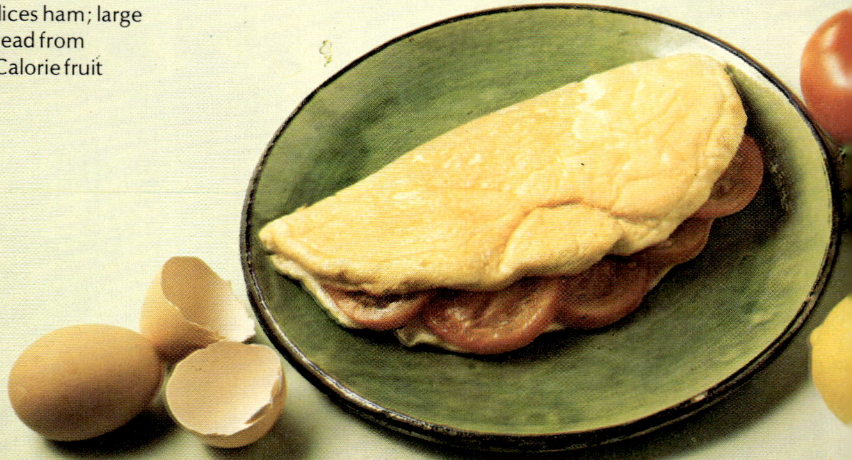

Lunch: Prawn salad; bread and butter from allowance; 50 Calorie fruit portion.
Supper: Thinly-sliced liver tossed in a little oil, served with sauce of yogurt and paprika; grilled tomatoes and mushrooms; cabbage; 50 Calorie fruit portion (p.11); tea or coffee with milk from allowance.

DAY FOUR
Breakfast: Beauty drink: whisk together small carton natural yogurt with the juice of 1 fresh orange and 1 egg; toast and butter from allowance; tea or coffee with milk from allowance.
Lunch: Small carton cottage cheese on bed of lettuce topped with sliced grapefruit and orange; bread and butter from allowance; tea or coffee from allowance.
Supper: 2 slices lean ham; large green salad; bread and butter from allowance; baked apple with raisins; tea or coffee with milk from allowance.

DAY FIVE
Breakfast: Orange juice; 2 eggs, scrambled with bread and butter from allowance; tea or coffee from allowance.
Lunch: Small cube hard cheese on toast (from allowance) or as open sandwich. Top with watercress, tomato and surround with more watercress; 50 Calorie fruit portion (p.11).
Supper: Chicken leg marinated in lemon juice and grilled; spinach; grilled tomato; fruit salad; bread and butter from allowance; tea or coffee with milk from allowance.

DAY SIX
Breakfast: Small portion unsweetened muesli with chopped apple and nuts on top; milk from allowance; 50 Calorie fruit portion (p.11); tea or coffee with milk from allowance.
Lunch: Sardines ($\frac{1}{2}$ small can) on toast from allowance; celery, cucumber and apple salad tossed in lemon juice; tea or coffee with milk from allowance.
Supper: Lean lamb chop; braised leeks and grilled tomatoes; small cube hard cheese with bread and butter from allowance; tea or coffee.

DAY SEVEN
Breakfast: Grapefruit juice; grilled kidneys on 1 slice bread or toast from allowance; 1 grilled tomato; tea or coffee with milk from allowance.
Lunch: Tuna fish sandwich (use bread slices from allowance and $\frac{1}{2}$ small tin tuna) with lemon juice and watercress; 50 Calorie fruit portion (p.11); tea or coffee with milk from allowance.
Supper: Veal escalope with wedge of lemon; salad of chicory, celery and orange tossed in orange juice; small natural yogurt with a few nuts and chopped dates stirred in; tea or coffee with milk from allowance.

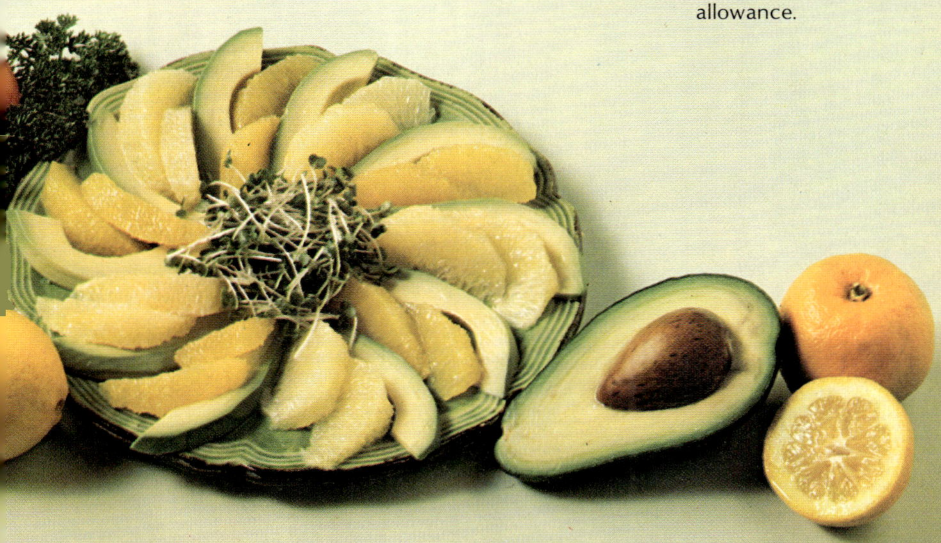

Quick weight-loss diet

Do you need to lose weight in a hurry for a holiday or special occasion? You can lose a lot of weight rapidly on the diet below: up to about 3.5 kg (7 lbs) in a week. However, the diet should not be followed for longer than that time, and you should make sure you are in good health before you start it. If in doubt, check with your doctor.

Although it cuts Calories drastically, the diet doesn't skimp on healthy foods such as fresh fruits, lean meat, fish and fresh vegetables. It does allow mid-morning and mid-afternoon snacks to take the edge off your appetite and encourage quick weight-loss. It's been proved that small, frequent meals are more efficient for rapid weight-loss than the same number of Calories consumed at one or two heavier meals. So don't cut the snacks out or eat them at the wrong time. Being caught off-guard without a suitable low-Calorie nibble is dangerous for even the most determined dieters; that's the time when you're most tempted to abandon the diet and buy a bar of chocolate or a hamburger. So make sure you have an airtight polythene bowl of vegetables, washed and cut into bite-sized pieces, with you at all times. The lunches are all packable: take your own picnic to work or if you go out.

The suppers are suitable for all the family if you add extras such as bread, potatoes and root vegetables. However, this diet is so stringent that you may have to exercise a lot of self-control to stop yourself joining in the extras. If this happens, try to eat your meal alone.

Finally, try to make sure you don't put back on all the weight you've lost when you finish the diet. Switch to a sensible eating plan such as the Health and beauty diet on p.18.

About 800 Calories

Daily allowance:
300ml ($\frac{1}{2}$ pint) skimmed milk; 7.5g ($\frac{1}{4}$oz) butter; bowl of raw vegetables for nibbling.

DAY ONE

Breakfast: Boiled egg, starch-reduced crispbread with butter from allowance; tea or coffee with milk from allowance.

Mid-morning: 50 Calorie fruit portion (p.11). Tea or coffee with milk from allowance.

Lunch: Slimmers' soup; bread from allowance; 1 slice ham; 50 Calorie fruit portion (p.11). Tea or coffee with milk from allowance.

Mid-afternoon: Unsweetened fruit juice; small portion tomato and mushroom salad with lemon juice dressing.

Supper: Grilled plaice; runner beans and grilled tomato; tea or coffee with milk from allowance.

DAY TWO

Breakfast: Medium-sized bowl fruit salad with unsweetened yogurt poured over; tea or

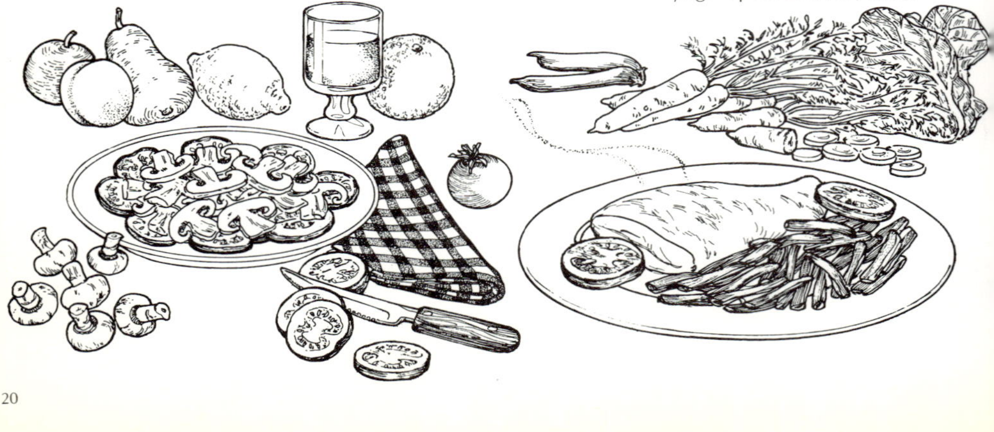

coffee with milk from allowance.
Mid-morning: 2.5cm (1″) cube hard cheese; bread from allowance; tea or coffee with milk from allowance.
Lunch: Half grapefruit (with sweetener); 2 slices cold chicken with large mixed salad and lemon juice dressing; tea or coffee with milk from allowance.
Mid-afternoon: 50 Calorie fruit portion (p.11).
Supper: Slimmers' soup; cauliflower with sauce made from yogurt, mustard and 2.5cm (1″) cube grated cheese heated together gently. Tea or coffee.

DAY THREE
Breakfast: Grilled mushrooms on toast from bread allowance; tea or coffee with milk from allowance.
Mid-morning: 50 Calorie fruit portion (p.11); tea or coffee.
Lunch: Cottage cheese American salad (p.50); tea or coffee with milk from allowance.
Mid-afternoon: Bowl of mixed fruit salad.
Supper: Chinese pork with bean shoots (p.50); 50 Calorie fruit portion (p.11); tea or coffee.

DAY FOUR
Breakfast: Poached egg on bed of spinach; tea or coffee with milk from allowance.
Mid-morning: Sliced tomato sandwich ($\frac{1}{2}$ round of bread from allowance).
Lunch: 1 slice ham with large mixed salad (lemon juice dressing); tea or coffee with milk from allowance.
Mid-afternoon: 50 Calorie fruit portion (p.11).
Supper: Cod fillet cooked in foil with mushrooms, tomatoes and chives; broccoli; tea or coffee with milk from allowance.

DAY FIVE
Breakfast: Small portion unsweetened muesli with sliced banana on top; tea or coffee with milk from allowance.
Mid-morning: Hard-boiled egg; 1 tomato; tea or coffee.
Lunch: Soup; Cottage cheese American salad (p.50); tea or coffee.
Mid-afternoon: 50 Calorie fruit portion (p.11).
Supper: 2 slices lean roast chicken; large portion cabbage or spinach; courgettes or braised celery; tea or coffee with milk from allowance.

DAY SIX
Breakfast: Small dish prunes with yogurt and nuts on top; toast from allowance with butter and beef extract. Tea or coffee.
Mid-morning: 2.5cm (1″) cube hard cheese with 1 crispbread (starch-reduced); tea or coffee.
Lunch: Hard-boiled egg with watercress, and mixture of sliced raw vegetables plus yogurt, mustard and chopped caper dip (pack in airtight plastic container to take to work).
Mid-afternoon: 50 Calorie fruit portion (p.11).
Supper: Small portion liver with orange sauce (squeeze $\frac{1}{4}$ orange into the gravy and decorate liver with sliced orange); cabbage; tea or coffee with milk from allowance.

DAY SEVEN
Breakfast: Poached egg on toast (from allowance); tea or coffee with milk from allowance.
Mid-morning: Glass of orange juice; small banana.
Lunch: Slimmers' soup; prawn salad (large mixed salad, prawns, lemon juice dressing); tea or coffee.
Mid-afternoon: 50 Calorie fruit portion (p.11).
Supper: 2 slices lean cold meat; jacket potato; peas; tea or coffee.

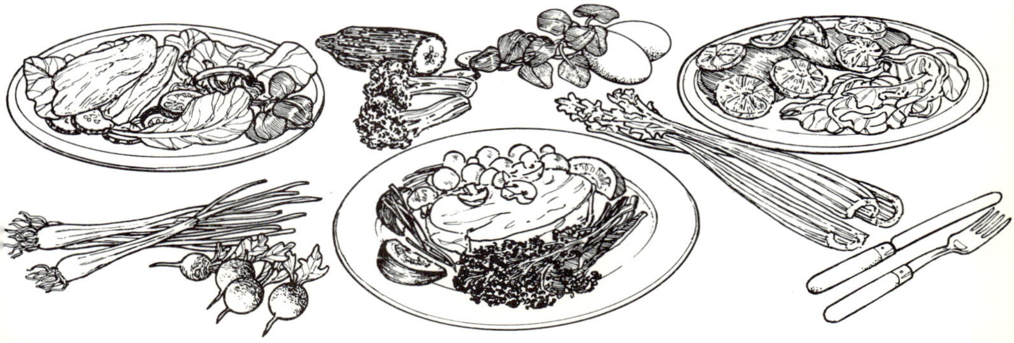

Wine diet

If you love good wine; there's no reason why you shouldn't enjoy it and get slim at the same time. You can lose weight *and* eat and drink really well on this diet. Dry red and white wine supplies 90 Calories a glass: about the same as a boiled sweet and much more enjoyable! So, it's quite possible to drink half a bottle a day (that's the generous allowance given) and still leave room in your diet for nutritious foods.

Expect a slow-but-sure weight-loss of about 1kg (2lbs) a week. The diet is ideal if you enjoy entertaining, as two of the evening meals consist of gourmet dishes cooked with wine. It is safe to follow for as long as you need to.

About 1500 Calories

Daily allowance:
300ml ($\frac{1}{2}$ pint) fresh whole milk for use in tea or coffee; 2 slices wholewheat bread; 15g ($\frac{1}{2}$ oz) butter; $\frac{1}{2}$ bottle dry white or red wine (*in addition* to wine used in recipes).

DAY ONE

Breakfast: 2 lamb's kidneys, grilled; 1 tomato grilled; bread or toast and butter from allowance; tea or coffee with milk from allowance.

Lunch: 2-egg omelette; green salad with lemon juice dressing; 50 Calorie fruit portion (p.11); tea or coffee (or wine allowance).

Supper: Veal paprika (p.52); broccoli or spinach; stewed apple with a little cream on top; wine allowance; tea or coffee with milk from allowance.

DAY TWO

Breakfast: Small grilled kipper with 1 slice bread and butter from allowance; tea or coffee.

Lunch: Half grapefruit, grilled with cinnamon on top; grilled mushrooms on 1 slice bread from allowance; 50 Calorie fruit portion (p.11); tea, coffee or wine from allowance.

Supper: Grilled lamb chop with sauce made from tinned tomatoes, herbs, garlic and a splash of dry red wine; large

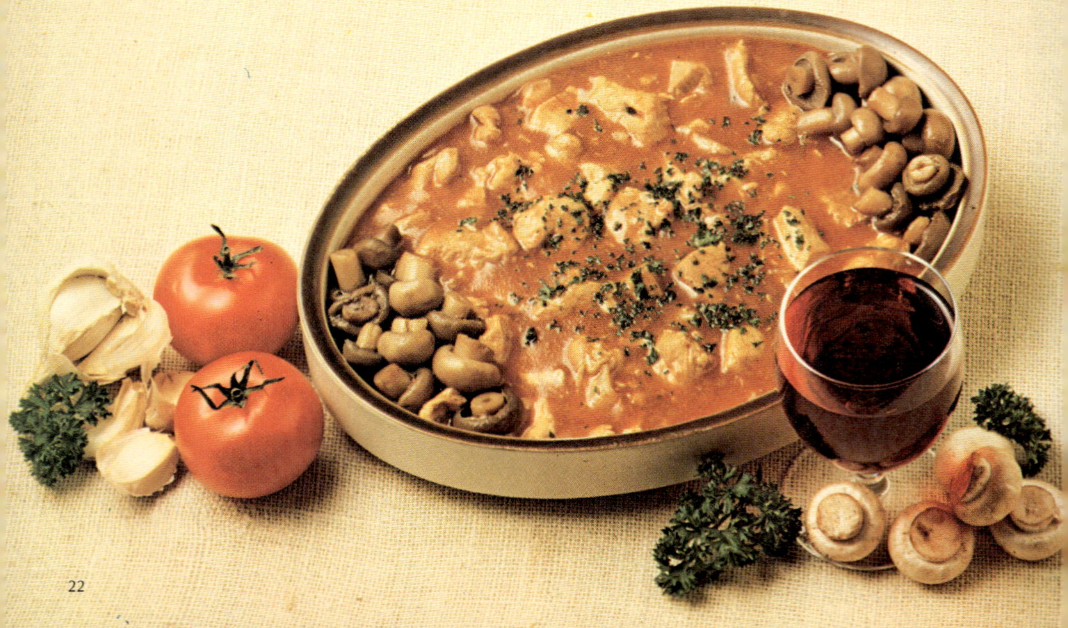

mixed salad; frozen mousse; wine allowance; tea or coffee with milk from allowance.

DAY THREE

Breakfast: Cold pear poached in wine; small piece cheese; bread and butter from allowance; tea or coffee.

Lunch: 2-egg herb omelette with green salad and lemon juice dressing; fresh fruit salad; wine from allowance; tea or coffee.

Supper: Lobster bisque with a dash of brandy; bread and butter from allowance; cottage cheese salad (generous portion of salad); wine from allowance; tea or coffee with milk from allowance.

DAY FOUR

Breakfast: Glass orange juice mixed with sparkling wine; 1 boiled egg; bread and butter from allowance; tea or coffee.

Lunch: Small slice quiche Lorraine; mixed salad with lemon juice dressing; wine from allowance; tea or coffee.

Supper: Mushrooms à la Grèque (stewed with tomatoes, onion, garlic, bay leaf and dry white wine); small helping grilled gammon; tomatoes; watercress; wine allowance; tea or coffee.

DAY FIVE

Breakfast: 2 rashers lean bacon; grilled tomato; bread and butter from allowance; tea or coffee.

Lunch: Hot beef extract drink with dash of dry sherry; selection of raw vegetables with dip of natural yogurt, horse-radish sauce, lemon juice and parsley.

Supper: Chicken livers cooked in red wine with stock and onions; small helping rice; wine allowance; tea or coffee.

DAY SIX

Breakfast: Red fruit salad with a dash of red wine and artificial sweetener (use raspberries, strawberries, red currants, plums etc. in season); bread and butter from allowance; tea or coffee.

Lunch: 50g (2oz) hard cheese on toast from allowance; 50 Calorie fruit portion (p.11); wine from allowance; tea or coffee.

Supper: Chicken leg marinated in lemon juice served with watercress; a little mashed potato; green salad with lemon juice; 50 Calorie fruit portion (p.11); wine from allowance; tea or coffee.

DAY SEVEN

Breakfast: Scrambled egg on 1 slice toast from allowance; large glass orange juice; tea or coffee with milk from allowance.

Lunch: 2 slices lean ham; mixed salad with lemon juice dressing; 50 Calorie fruit portion (p.11); wine from allowance; tea or coffee.

Supper: Beef ragout in red wine (p.52); cabbage; carrots; fresh fruit salad; wine from allowance; tea or coffee.

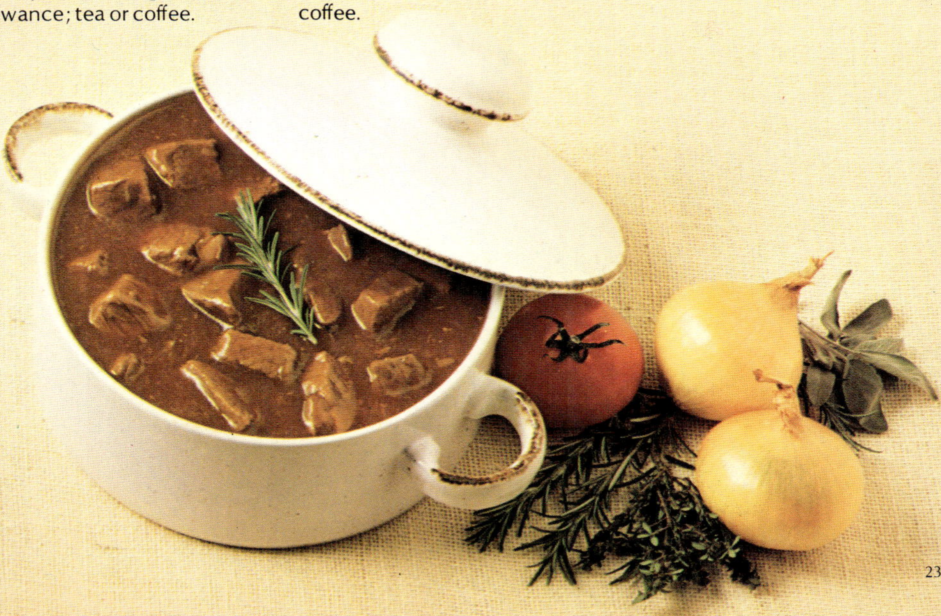

Anti-stress diet

If you feel nervous, irritable and depressed most of the time then you may be suffering from stress. This 20th-century disease is unfortunately becoming increasingly common amongst housewives as well as superstars and nutritionists are convinced that our bad eating habits certainly aren't helping us cope with it.

The first essential when you feel under par and under stress is a good balanced diet. However, even a balanced diet may be short on anti-stress nutrients like the B complex vitamins (especially thiamine and vitamin B6 in yeast, wheatgerm and liver, and B12, which has its richest source in liver but also occurs in yeast extract. The diet below allows for all these things while cutting out alcohol and high-carbohydrate junk foods which do nothing to adequately nourish the body or brain.

Follow the diet for as long as you need to and combine it with an exercise course chosen from the three that begin on p.44. Physical exertion is often the best remedy for mental exhaustion. However, if you feel fragile and tetchy, do start with the gentle exercises and gradually work your way up to the more strenuous ones. Set aside some time each day for your exercises and try to include regular walking, swimming or jogging in your fitness plan. Frequent short holidays are often more relaxing than one long one.

About 1200 Calories
Daily allowance:
300 ml ($\frac{1}{2}$ pint) milk for use in tea or coffee; 6g ($\frac{1}{4}$oz) butter or margarine.

DAY ONE
Breakfast: Small bowl breakfast cereal with wheatgerm on top; milk (in addition to allowance); tea or coffee.
Lunch: Large mixed salad with 50g (2oz) grated cheese and wheatgerm on top; tea or coffee.
Supper: Beef and kidney ring with buttered corn (p.50); green vegetables; 1 small potato.

DAY TWO
Breakfast: Poached egg on 1 slice toast with butter from allowance; unsweetened fruit juice; tea or coffee.

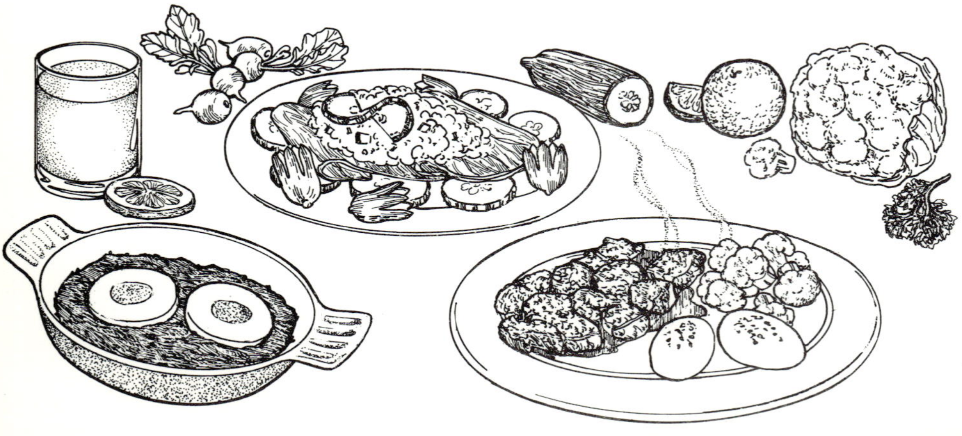

Lunch: 50g (2oz) ham topped with 100g (4oz) cottage cheese mixed with 1 tsp chives, $1\frac{1}{2}$ tbs wheatgerm, 1 tbs chopped cucumber, salt and pepper and garnished with radishes and cucumber; tea or coffee.
Supper: Grilled herring with mustard butter (p.50); broccoli.

DAY THREE
Breakfast: Unsweetened muesli with wheatgerm on top; milk (in addition to allowance); tea or coffee.
Lunch: Spinach topped with 2 poached eggs; tea or coffee.
Supper: 200g ($\frac{1}{2}$ lb) lean stewing steak, coated with wheatgerm and flour, fried and then stewed for $2\frac{1}{2}$ hours in a little pale ale and seasoning; cauliflower; 2 new potatoes.

DAY FOUR
Breakfast: Small bowl breakfast cereal with wheatgerm on top and milk (in addition to allowance); unsweetened orange juice; tea or coffee.
Lunch: Half a small can of tuna fish on large mixed salad sprinkled with wheatgerm; 1 slice wholewheat bread and butter from allowance; tea or coffee.
Supper: Lean pork chop; cauliflower; cabbage; grilled tomatoes; 2 small boiled potatoes; tea or coffee.

DAY FIVE
Breakfast: 1 slice wholemeal toast with butter from allowance and honey; fruit juice (unsweetened); tea or coffee.
Lunch: 50g (2oz) grated cheese; hard-boiled egg with green salad and lemon juice dressing.
Supper: 150g (6oz) plaice fillet cooked in the oven with mushrooms, 1 small grated onion, 1 tbs water and lemon juice for 30 minutes; 1 jacket potato; tea or coffee.

DAY SIX
Breakfast: Small portion muesli topped with wheatgerm; fruit juice; tea or coffee.
Lunch: 2-egg omelette with wheatgerm, chopped parsley and onion filling; 1 slice wholewheat bread and butter from allowance.
Supper: 75g (3oz) (raw weight) spaghetti with sauce of 100g (4oz) minced beef, a little tomato puree, seasoning and tobasco to taste; large green salad with lemon juice dressing.

DAY SEVEN
Breakfast: 1 boiled egg; 1 slice wholewheat bread with butter from allowance; fruit juice; tea or coffee.
Lunch: Home-made tomato soup: use a small can tomatoes, stock, garlic and chopped onion simmered and blended together; roast chicken; cauliflower; 2 small boiled potatoes; orange salad with 2 chopped dates.
Supper: Fresh fruit salad with yogurt and wheatgerm topping.

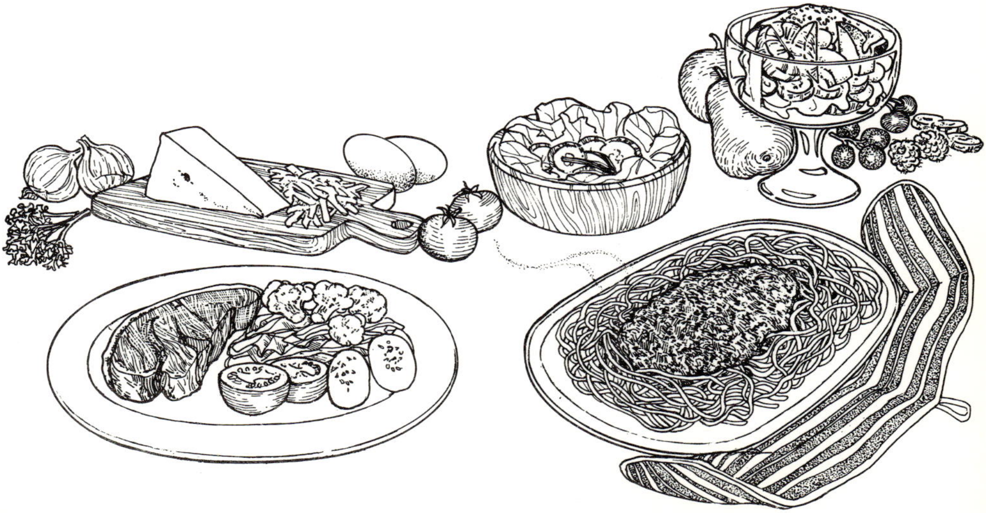

Low cholesterol diet

There is reasonable evidence that high levels of cholesterol in the blood contribute to coronary heart disease. For this reason, some people are advised by their doctors to reduce the fat content of their diet. Cut Calories as well and you will be safeguarding against obesity, another well known contributor to some heart conditions.

Avoid fat on meat, in gravies, sauces, pastry, biscuits, mayonnaise and cakes. Replace hard cheese with Edam or cottage cheese and cream with yogurt. Use skimmed milk instead of full milk and polyunsaturated fat and margarine instead of butter. Cut down on high cholesterol foods such as eggs, offal and seafood. Regular gentle exercise will help lower blood cholesterol levels as well as keep you trim. But *check with your doctor first.*

About 1200 Calories

Daily allowance:
300ml ($\frac{1}{2}$ pint) skimmed milk for use in tea or coffee; 2 slices wholemeal bread; 15g ($\frac{1}{2}$oz) polyunsaturated margarine.
Alcohol: $\frac{1}{2}$ pint beer or 1 short drink with low-Calorie mixers.

DAY ONE

Breakfast: 1 glass orange juice; 1 slice bread from allowance with margarine, cottage cheese and tomato; tea or coffee.
Lunch: Grilled white fish; mixed salad with a little vegetable oil and vinegar dressing; 50 Calorie fruit portion (p.11); tea or coffee.
Supper: Minced beef and onion curry; 1 tbs rice; orange and date salad; tea or coffee.

DAY TWO

Breakfast: Orange and grapefruit segments; grilled mushrooms on bread and margarine from allowance; tea or coffee.
Lunch: 2 slices chicken; broccoli spears; grilled tomatoes; tea or coffee.
Supper: Fish pie, mixed vegetable salad with vegetable oil and vinegar dressing; tea or coffee.

DAY THREE

Breakfast: Slice of cold lean ham; tomato; bread or toast from allowance; tea or coffee.

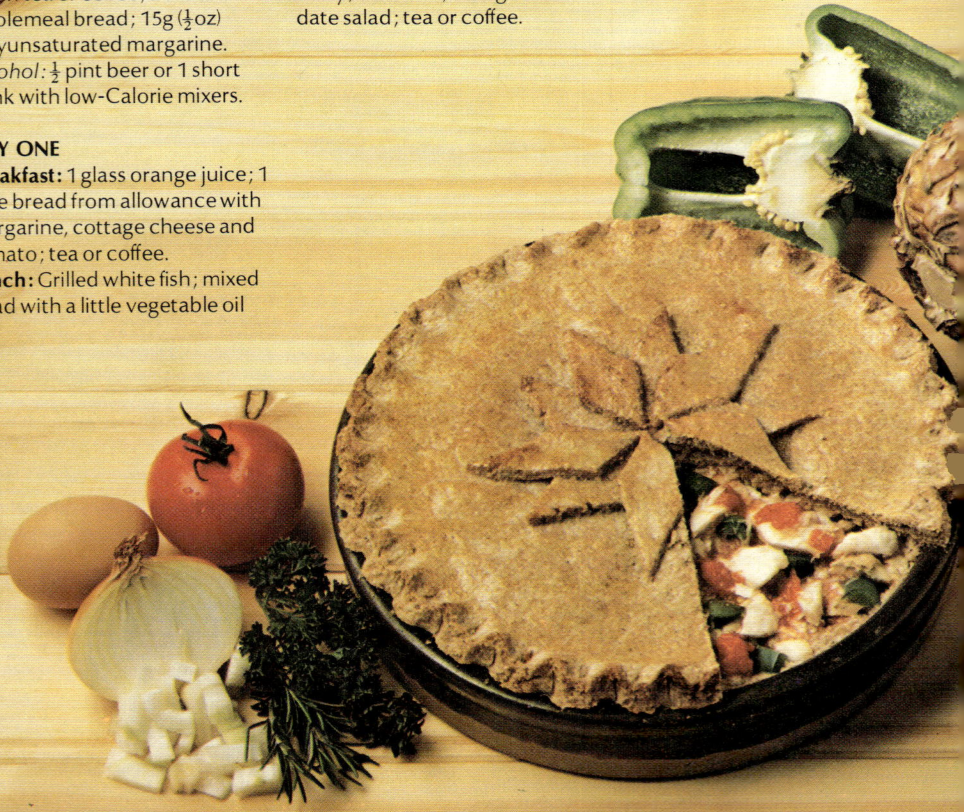

Lunch: Cottage cheese salad; bread and margarine from allowance; tea or coffee.
Supper: Melon, cucumber and tomato salad with lemon and thyme dressing; lean steak with courgettes; tea or coffee.

DAY FOUR
Breakfast: Stewed apple with artificial sweetener; natural yogurt; bread and margarine from allowance; tea or coffee.
Lunch: 2 slices lean ham; mixed salad with lemon juice and vegetable oil dressing; 50 Calorie fruit portion (p.11); tea or coffee.
Supper: Mixed vegetable casserole with yogurt topping; Pineapple crunch (p.52); tea or coffee.

DAY FIVE
Breakfast: Small poached haddock; grilled tomato; bread and margarine from allowance; tea or coffee.
Lunch: Lean lamb chop; 1 small potato; cauliflower; tea or coffee.
Supper: Chilled cucumber soup; bread and margarine from allowance; chicken slices with green salad and lemon dressing; 50 Calorie fruit portion (p.11); tea or coffee.

DAY SIX
Breakfast: Small bowl of muesli with apple on top; milk from allowance; toast from allowance with beef extract; tea or coffee.
Lunch: Large American salad using cottage cheese, fruit (such as pear or peach) on a bed of lettuce; tea or coffee.
Supper: Moussaka with lean minced beef and yogurt topping; fresh fruit salad; tea or coffee.

DAY SEVEN
Breakfast: $\frac{1}{2}$ grapefruit; grilled tomatoes on slice of toast from allowance, topped with grated Edam; tea or coffee.
Lunch: 2 slices lean roast beef; sprouts or broccoli; carrots; fruit fool made with any 50 Calorie fruit portion (p.11) mixed with yogurt; tea or coffee.
Supper: Cold roast beef open sandwich with remainder of bread allowance decorated with watercress and gherkins; tea or coffee.

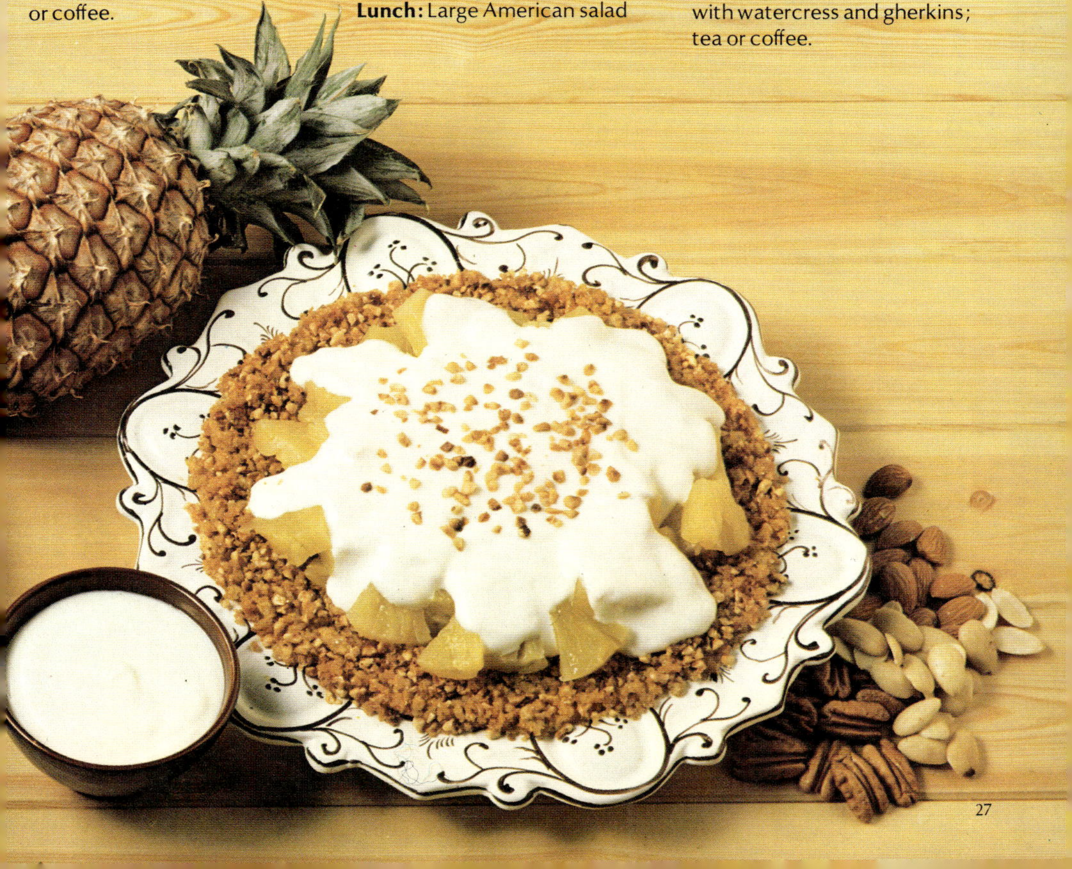

High fibre diet

Recently, wide publicity has been given to the importance of adequate fibre in the diet to prevent a whole range of diseases such as diverticulitis, bowel cancer, heart disease and gall-bladder disease. But adequate fibre, the scaffolding that supports plant cells, can also be important for slimmers.

High-fibre foods (such as raw fruit, vegetables, bran, wholewheat bread, brown rice) are more satisfying and bulky and therefore encourage slimmers to stay the course on a high-fibre diet. Experts also point out that there is now evidence that fibre actually prevents small quantities of energy being absorbed from the intestine and that fibre-eaters excrete more fat in their stools than those on a low-fibre diet.

If you have a history of constipation, dental caries and a sluggish stomach, then a high-fibre diet is a good idea. However, some fibre-rich foods (such as wholewheat bread, brown rice) are also high in Calories, so you certainly won't lose weight if you simply add lots of fibre-rich foods to your diet.

The diet below includes fibre-rich items such as bran, raw fruits, vegetables, wholewheat bread and brown rice, but it is also Calorie-controlled to ensure a steady weight-loss. You'll find it very satisfying, although you may feel a bit 'windy' at first. It's safe to follow for as long as neccessary, but it isn't recommended if your bowel motions are already a bit too regular for comfort. If in doubt, check with your doctor.

To help increase the fibre value and preserve nutrients in your day-to-day diet, follow these rules:

1 Avoid white flour and white flour products. Always look for wholewheat bread, flour and cakes or bake your own. (Not recommended for slimmers without much will-power as the gorgeous smell encourages you to eat too much.)
2 Serve fruit raw, with skins intact, and where possible serve vegetables raw or cooked in their skins in very little water. Steaming, pressure-cooking or grilling are the best methods or you can sauté vegetables, Chinese style, in a very little oil.
3 Cut down sugar.
4 Sprinkle bran on cereals, stir into soups and sprinkle on fruit dishes.

About 1200 Calories
Daily allowance:
300ml ($\frac{1}{2}$ pint) fresh whole milk for use on cereal and in tea or coffee; 3 slices wholewheat bread; 15g ($\frac{1}{2}$oz) butter.

DAY ONE
Breakfast: Small helping bran cereal with grated apple on top; milk from allowance; tea or coffee with milk from allowance.
Lunch: Hamburger steak on wholewheat bread from allowance; salad of grated white cabbage, carrot, yogurt and a little vinegar; 50 Calorie fruit portion (p.11); tea or coffee with milk from allowance.
Supper: Herring in oatmeal (p.54) with Brown rice and tomato salad (p.54); tea or coffee with milk from allowance; bread and butter from allowance.

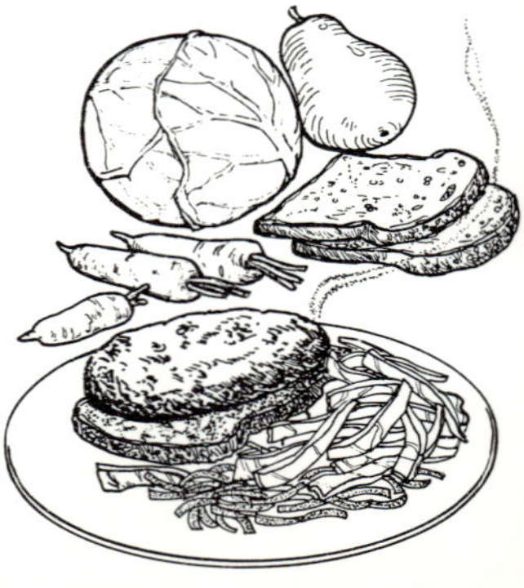

DAY TWO
Breakfast: Poached egg on bread from allowance; orange juice (unsweetened); tea or coffee with milk from allowance.
Lunch: Small portion tuna with green pepper, celery and cucumber salad in yogurt and lemon juice dressing; bread and butter from allowance; 50 Calorie fruit portion (p.11); tea or coffee.
Supper: Lamb chop (small, lean) with spinach, grilled tomatoes; stewed apple (sweetened with artificial sweetener) with crunchy oatmeal or bran topping; tea or coffee.

DAY THREE
Breakfast: Fresh fruit salad (leave skins on soft fruit, apples, pears) with yogurt and lemon topping; bread and butter from allowance; tea or coffee.
Lunch: 1 pilchard; 1 tomato stuffed with wholemeal breadcrumbs, chopped chives and grilled; 50 Calorie fruit portion (p.11); tea or coffee.
Supper: Small bowl lentil soup; large mixed salad with lemon juice dressing; bread and butter from allowance; tea or coffee.

DAY FOUR
Breakfast: Small helping bran cereal with sliced pear on top; milk from allowance; bread and butter from allowance; tea or coffee.
Lunch: 3 slices cooked chicken with chicory, cucumber and cashew nut salad; 50 Calorie fruit portion (p.11); tea or coffee.
Supper: Cod steak with 1 tbs brown rice and separate tomato and onion salad (lemon juice, herbs and garlic as dressing); tea or coffee.

DAY FIVE
Breakfast: Unsweetened muesli with grapes on top; milk from allowance; bread and butter from allowance; tea or coffee.
Lunch: Cheese salad: 25g (1oz) grated cheese on large mixed salad using raw vegetables such as cabbage, carrot, lettuce etc. with lemon juice dressing; 50 Calorie fruit portion (p.11); tea or coffee.
Supper: Tomato soup (use canned tomatoes with stock, oregano or basil) with wholemeal bread croutons (from allowance); minced beef with onions and cabbage; tea or coffee.

DAY SIX
Breakfast: Grapefruit juice; scrambled eggs (2) on wholemeal toast from allowance; tea or coffee.
Lunch: Tomato soup (as yesterday's supper); wholemeal bread, butter and 25g (1oz) cheese; tea or coffee.
Supper: Small piece of fillet steak with mushrooms, cucumber and apple salad; bread and butter from allowance (if left over!); baked apple stuffed with raisins; tea or coffee.

DAY SEVEN
Breakfast: Orange juice: 2 rashers bacon (grilled); toast from allowance; tea or coffee.
Lunch: Stuffed lamb (p.54); broccoli; fresh fruit salad (leave apple, pear skins *on*) with crispy bran sprinkled on top; tea or coffee.
Supper: Lamb chop (small, lean) with spinach, grilled tomatoes; stewed apple (sweetened with artificial sweetener) with crunchy oatmeal or bran topping; tea or coffee.

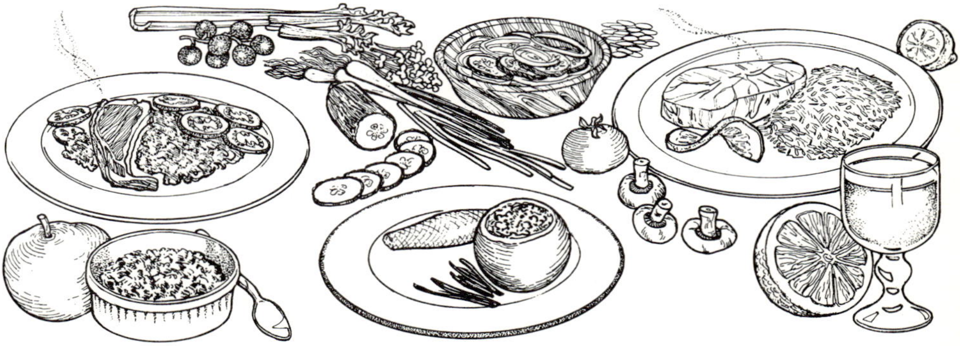

Vegetarian diet

Even if you are not a vegetarian, a non-meat diet can be fun (and beneficial for your health) to try occasionally. The main problem in vegetarian cooking is to ensure adequate supplies of protein: but this can be achieved by using yogurt, cheese, cereals and pulses such as lentils and haricot beans. However, when you're slimming, it's vital to limit the high-Calorie foods, so do beware of overdoing the cheese, cereals and pulses!
The diet below will help you slim quite rapidly: expect to lose about 1.5kg (3lbs) a week. Don't follow it for more than two weeks. Remember that really fresh, organically grown produce usually tastes extra delicious as well as being free from possible harmful chemicals. Shop around for the most appetising raw materials and add extra touches with home-grown herbs and salads.

1000-1200 Calories
Daily allowance:
300ml ($\frac{1}{2}$ pint) low-fat separated milk; 6g ($\frac{1}{4}$oz) butter.
Drinks: Unlimited water, mineral water, herbal tea made from an infusion of mint, camomile and rosehip, tea with milk from allowance or de-caffeinated coffee with milk from allowance.

DAY ONE
Breakfast: Small glass tomato juice; small bowl muesli topped with chopped apple and nuts; milk from allowance.
Lunch: Half avocado pear with 50g (2oz) cottage cheese on top; large mixed vegetable salad with lemon juice dressing.
Supper: Vegetable casserole with yogurt topping (p.53); fresh fruit.

DAY TWO
Breakfast: Small glass orange juice; 1 slice wholewheat bread with butter from allowance topped with 50g (2oz) cottage cheese.
Lunch: Apple, carrot and orange salad sprinkled with

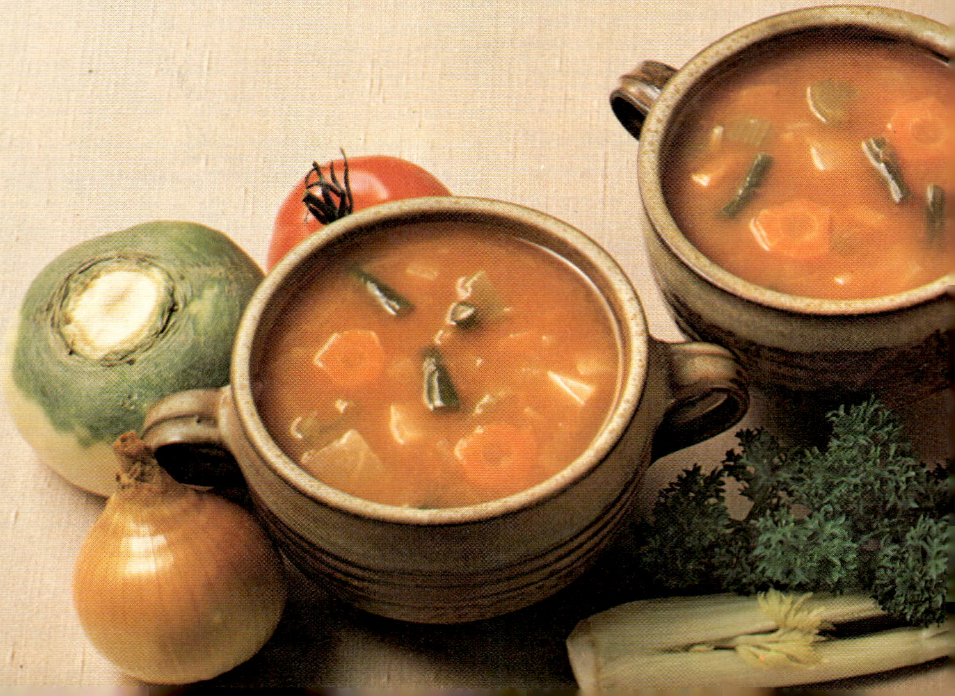

lemon juice and 50g (2oz) peanuts.
Supper: 200g (8oz) cooked brown rice mixed with chopped red and green pepper topped with 25g (1oz) grated cheese; 1 small banana.

DAY THREE
Breakfast: Small glass grapefruit juice; 2-egg fluffy omelette with 1 slice wholemeal bread and butter from allowance.
Lunch: Cucumber salad with mint, yogurt and lemon juice dressing; 50g (2oz) Cheddar cheese; handful of grapes.
Supper: Country vegetable soup (p.53); cauliflower cheese with 25g (1oz) grated Cheddar sprinkled on top; 1 slice wholewheat bread and butter from allowance.

DAY FOUR
Breakfast: Small glass carrot juice; slice of melon chopped and mixed with toasted almonds and pineapple cubes; natural yogurt.
Lunch: Chopped hard-boiled egg mixed with a little mustard and grated onion on a bed of lettuce garnished with salad vegetables.
Supper: Small green pepper stuffed with 200g (8oz) cooked brown rice mixed with chopped cooked carrot and onion and topped with 2 tbs yogurt; 1 orange.

DAY FIVE
Breakfast: Small glass mixed vegetable juice; poached egg on 1 slice wholewheat bread with butter from allowance.
Lunch: Chopped melon with cottage cheese and lemon juice dressing; fresh fruit salad.
Supper: Small bowl lentil soup; 1 slice wholewheat bread with butter from allowance; raw carrot sticks to nibble.

DAY SIX
Breakfast: Small glass orange juice; grilled mushrooms on 1 slice wholewheat toast with butter from allowance.
Lunch: Hard-boiled egg; starch-reduced crispbread with butter from allowance; 1 small banana.
Supper: Ratatouille (made with stewed onion, tomato, courgettes and very little oil) with 25g (1oz) cheese topping; 1 pear.

DAY SEVEN
Breakfast: Small glass grapefruit juice; poached egg on 1 slice wholewheat toast.
Lunch: Small portion Country vegetable soup (p.53); mixed vegetable salad platter with sauce of 2 tbs natural yogurt, egg yolk, mustard and a little grated parmesan.
Supper: Hot fruit compote; 1 slice wholewheat bread and butter from allowance; 25g (1oz) hard cheese.

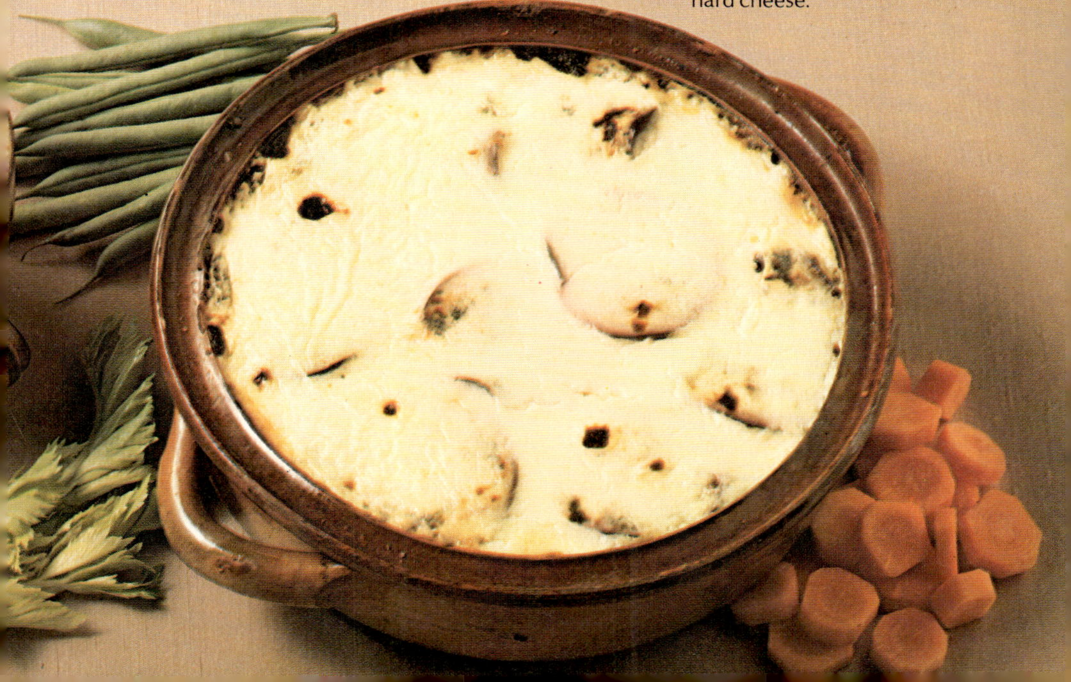

Pregnancy diet

An expectant mother needs to watch her diet very carefully indeed. She also needs to watch her weight, to avoid developing complications such as toxaemia, high blood pressure and labour problems. The weight-gain to aim for is around 11kg (22lbs): danger time for many mothers is when they start to put their feet up about half-way through the pregnancy. Suddenly, their weight starts shooting up and a stringent control is needed.

So it's best to think constructively about diet right from the very first months of your pregnancy. You need increased amounts of all the major nutrients, especially protein, calcium, iron and vitamins A and D. You don't need extra starches or sugary foods for energy.

Your diet should include a pint of milk a day, cheese, meat, (particularly liver and kidney), fish (especially oily fish such as herrings, kippers and sardines which are a good source of vitamin D for your baby's growth), fruit and vegetables. If you feel queasy during the early months, a late night milk and biscuit snack can help, as can a nibble of dry biscuit or crispbread during the day. If you literally can't keep a thing down you must see your doctor for vitamin supplements to ensure the baby's healthy development. However, early morning sickness and general nausea soon pass off after the first couple of months. Sometimes it can also help to take smaller meals more frequently as an empty tummy often leads to a feeling of nausea.

As the pregnancy develops, constipation can become a major problem. Increase the roughage (fresh fruit, vegetables, bran) in your diet but don't take laxatives such as liquid paraffin which may dissolve fat-soluble vitamins. Drink plenty of water.

What about cravings? Many overweight mothers-to-be use these as an excuse to indulge in cream cakes, fatty fried foods and chocolates. *Don't.* If you get a passion for fresh fruit, by all means indulge it, but do be sensible about the fatteners. Luckily, cravings often turn out to be highly nutritious although a bit odd: cheese and strawberries for instance or sliced avocados with scrambled egg!

About 1600 Calories

Daily allowance:
600ml (1 pint) milk and 1 sweet biscuit on waking.

DAY ONE

Breakfast: 1 boiled egg; 1 slice wholewheat bread and butter; 1 apple.
Lunch: 2 thin slices corned beef; salad of lettuce, tomato, sweetcorn; fruit yogurt.
Supper: Small pork chop; large helping cabbage or sprouts; 1 tbs carrots; baked apple stuffed with raisins.
Snacks: 2 dry biscuits for queasy moments!

DAY TWO

Breakfast: 25g (1oz) muesli or bran cereal topped with sliced banana and milk from allowance. 1 slice wholewheat toast with yeast extract.

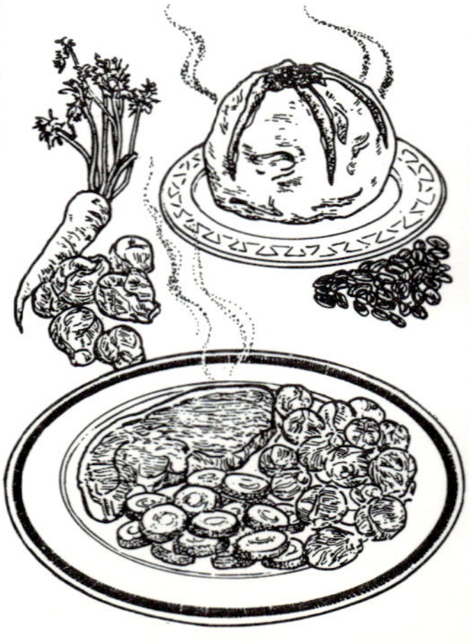

Lunch: 1 can slimmers' soup topped with 25g (1oz) grated Edam cheese; 1 slice wholewheat bread and butter; 1 orange.
Supper: 100g (4oz) thinly sliced liver sautéed in a little butter and served with 1 boiled onion; broccoli; 1 grilled tomato; fresh fruit salad.
Snacks: 2 small cheese biscuits.

DAY THREE
Breakfast: 1 small fillet poached haddock; 1 slice wholewheat bread and butter.
Lunch: Half grapefruit; open sandwich of 1 slice wholewheat bread topped with 2 tbs cottage cheese and orange segments.
Supper: 150g (6oz) minced beef cooked with chopped onion and carrot and topped with 25g (1oz) grated cheese. Large mixed salad with low-Calorie dressing.

DAY FOUR
Breakfast: 1 rasher lean bacon, grilled with mushrooms and 1 tomato; 1 slice wholewheat bread and butter.
Lunch: Mix 50g (2oz) chopped mixed nuts with 1 chopped apple and 50g (2oz) cottage cheese. Serve on bed of lettuce; 1 pear.
Supper: 100g (4oz) grilled kidney with mushrooms; 1 tbs carrots; cabbage; 1 fruit yogurt.
Snacks: 2 crispbreads with beef extract spread.

DAY FIVE
Breakfast: 1 small slice melon; 25g (1oz) any cereal with milk from allowance; 1 slice wholewheat bread, butter and marmalade.
Lunch: 100g (4oz) tuna fish; large mixed salad with low-Calorie dressing; 1 orange.
Supper: Dutch peppers (p.55); 50g (2oz) boiled rice; 1 apple.
Snacks: 1 dry biscuit.

DAY SIX
Breakfast: 1 boiled egg; 1 slice wholewheat bread and butter.
Lunch: Tangy salmon avocado (p.55); small glass orange juice.
Supper: 100g (4oz) beef stew with carrots; cabbage or sprouts; 25g (1oz) hard cheese with 1 cream cracker.
Snacks: 2 sweet biscuits.

DAY SIX (alternative)
Breakfast: 2 eggs, scrambled with a little butter and milk from allowance on 1 slice wholemeal toast topped with 25g (1oz) grated Edam cheese melted under the grill.
Lunch: 2 thin slices ham with large mixed salad and low-Calorie dressing.
Supper: Haddock scallops (p.55); broccoli; 1 grilled tomato.
Snacks: 2 small cheese biscuits.

DAY SEVEN
Breakfast: 25g (1oz) muesli with milk from allowance; 1 slice wholewheat toast and butter; 1 orange.
Lunch: 2 slices lean roast meat; courgettes; cabbage; 1 small potato.
Supper: Small grilled herring; 1 slice wholewheat bread and butter.
Snacks: 1 dry biscuit or 2 small cheese biscuits.

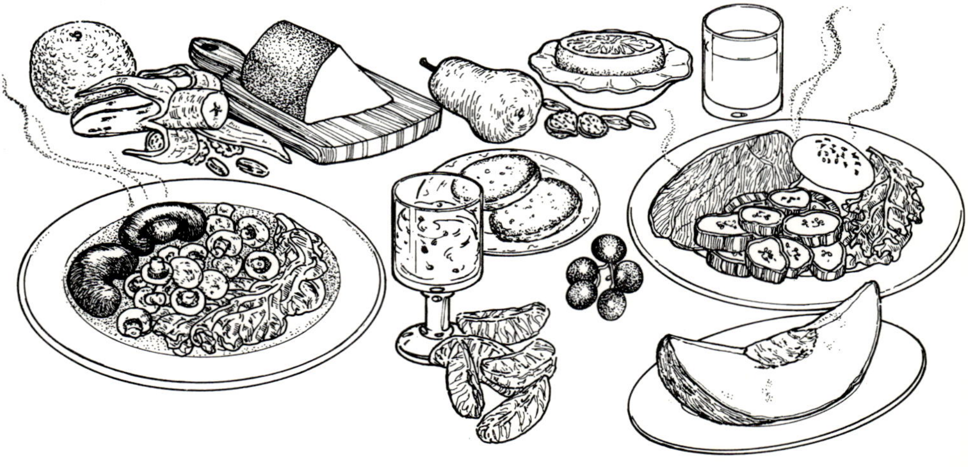

Post-natal diet

Every woman wants to regain her pre-baby shape as quickly as possible after the birth. But, it's also vital to make sure you are properly nourished to cope with the extra demands on your time and energy that a small baby brings. If you are breast-feeding, you need extra fluids as well as a nourishing diet, but you will lose around 600 Calories a day, so getting back into shape should be much easier for you. The diet below provides much-needed nutrients like protein and calcium. It's not *too* strict: you can swap the lunches and suppers and there's a tasty, sustaining snack which you can eat any time (day or night!) when your energy is flagging. The main meals on days 3 and 6 are a bit more special so make these evenings an occasion for yourself and your husband. Allow time for a treat during the first busy weeks at home: visit the hairdresser or get a friend to give you a beauty treatment.

NB Breastfeeding mothers should choose low-fat milk and top up their fluid intake with low-Calorie drinks, water, tea or coffee.

Daily allowance:
300 ml ($\frac{1}{2}$ pint) whole milk or 600ml (1 pint) low-fat separated milk.

DAY ONE

Breakfast: 25g (1oz) any breakfast cereal; 150ml ($\frac{1}{4}$ pint) milk (in addition to daily allowance) topped with sliced apple, small banana or 1 tbs sultanas.

Light meal: Thicken 300ml ($\frac{1}{2}$ pint) chicken stock with 1 heaped tsp flour and add 75g (3oz) chopped chicken and sprinkling of mixed herbs or chopped chives. Heat through and season; 25g (1oz) slice of bread with 7g ($\frac{1}{4}$oz) butter; apple or orange.

Main meal: Brown an average sized lean lamb chop under the grill, place in casserole topped with onion and tomato slices and 75ml ($\frac{1}{8}$ pint) seasoned stock. Top with a mixture of 25g (1oz) grated Edam cheese and 15g ($\frac{1}{2}$oz) fresh breadcrumbs. Cover and cook in a slow oven for 1$\frac{1}{2}$ hours and eat with a small boiled potato, green beans and carrots. 1 natural yogurt.

Snack: Make a white sauce with 2 tbs milk, 1 level tbs cornflour and mix with 25g (4oz) Edam cheese and 1 level tsp mustard powder. Add black pepper to taste, chopped chives, onion or gherkin and use a little of the spread to top a slice of bread (toast it if you like). The rest will be for your snack on other weekdays. Use it as a 'mum reviver' when your energy is flagging!

DAY TWO

Breakfast: 1 whole fruit yogurt with 1 banana and 1 tbs sultanas.

Light meal: 65g (2$\frac{1}{2}$oz) lean cold ham with salad of 25g (1oz)

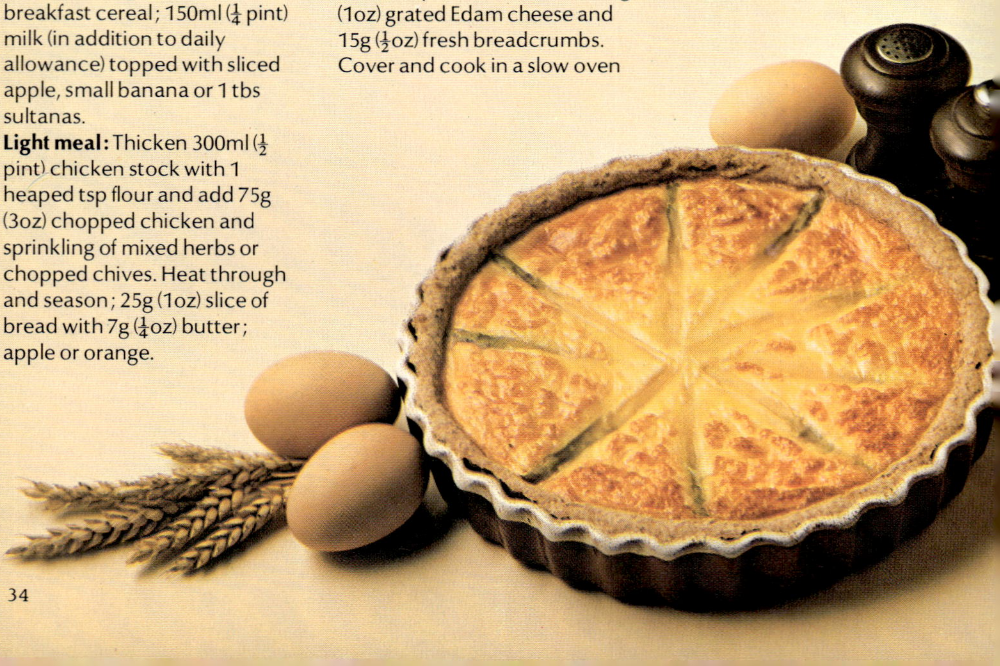

grated hard cheese, 45g ($1\frac{3}{4}$oz) shredded raw red cabbage, 15g ($\frac{1}{2}$oz) peanuts, $\frac{1}{2}$ apple cored and chopped, lemon juice to taste.
Main meal: 150g (6oz) filleted cod covered with parsley sauce made from 15g ($\frac{1}{2}$oz) butter, 15g ($\frac{1}{2}$oz) flour and 150ml ($\frac{1}{4}$ pint) milk (in addition to your allowance), seasoning, chopped parsley; small boiled potato, spinach or broccoli; 1 banana.
Snack: 'Mum reviver'!

DAY THREE
Breakfast: Small glass fruit juice; 1 egg boiled; 1 slice bread with scraping of butter.
Light meal: 2 small sausages, grilled, with small boiled potato; small portion of peas; 2 tbs thin gravy.
Main meal: Cheese and asparagus flan (p.56).
Snack: Apple or orange.

DAY FOUR
Breakfast: 2 rashers bacon, grilled, with 1 tomato served on 1 slice toast with scraping of butter.
Light meal: 2-egg omelette cooked in a little butter with 40g ($1\frac{1}{2}$oz) hard cheese grated as filling. Salad with lemon juice dressing.
Main meal: Fry 2 rashers bacon and use their fat to fry 125g (4oz) liver. Serve with green beans or carrots, medium boiled potato, 2 tbs thin gravy; 1 apple or orange.
Snack: 'Mum reviver'.

DAY FIVE
Breakfast: Small portion any cereal with 150ml ($\frac{1}{4}$ pint) milk (in addition to allowance), 1 sliced apple, small banana or 1 tbs sultanas.
Light meal: 75g (3oz) roast chicken with red cabbage salad (as Day two).
Main meal: Spaghetti Bolognaise: 25g (1oz) raw spaghetti with 75g (3oz) lean mince and 300ml ($\frac{1}{2}$ pint) beef stock, tomato slices, 50g (2oz) grated Edam.
Snack: 'Mum reviver'.

DAY SIX
Breakfast: Small glass fruit juice; 1 egg poached on 1 slice bread with scraping of butter.
Light meal: Corned beef hash: heat 50g (2oz) chopped corned beef with a tomato sauce made from 4 tbs stock heated with 2 level tsp seasoned cornflour, 2 finely chopped tomatoes and mixed herbs. Serve with small boiled potato, cabbage or green beans.
Main meal: Fish supreme (p.56).
Snack: 'Mum reviver'.

DAY SEVEN
Breakfast: Small kipper grilled with a little butter and a slice of bread with scraping of butter.
Light meal: 1 egg, poached and served on a bed of spinach tossed in a little butter, topped with 50g (2oz) grated hard cheese, browned under the grill; 1 apple or orange.
Main meal: 100g (4oz) lean roast beef, lamb or pork; medium roast potato; green beans or carrots, 2 tbs thin gravy.

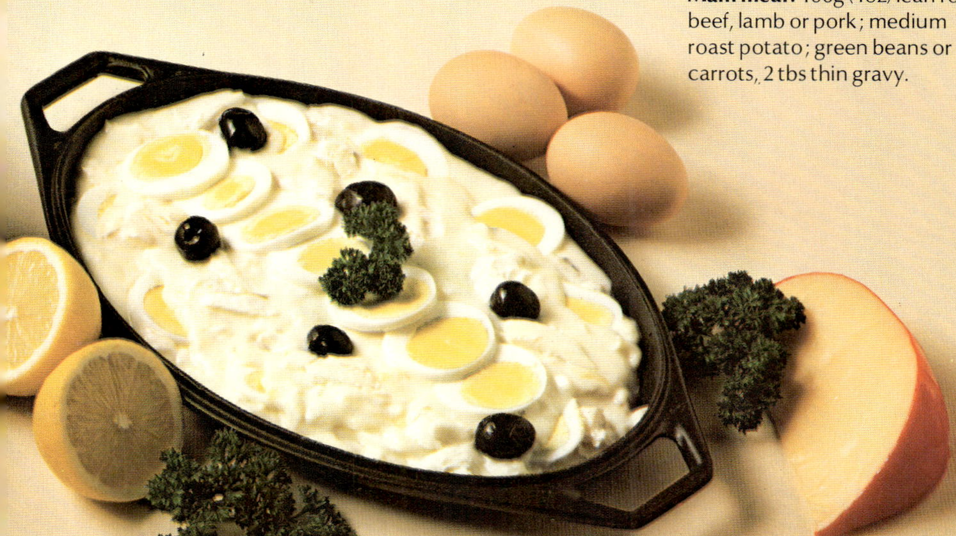

Babies' diet

You will get your baby off to a good slim start in life if you breast-feed. Human milk is convenient, the perfect formula, the right temperature and free from infection. There is also evidence that breast-fed babies learn to judge satiety more quickly than those who are given a set quantity from a bottle.

If you do bottle-feed, make sure you prepare the formula correctly. If it's too thick (and many mothers believe in adding an extra scoop of milk powder), your baby will take in too much salt and possibly become obese. Recent studies show that fat babies stand every chance of becoming fat adults. Remember when you're at the clinic that babies should be checked for length as well as weight regularly to give a balanced picture of development.

Don't forget that babies get thirsty as well as hungry. Many crying babies are given an extra bottle of milk when cooled boiled water would have been just as welcome.

Once weaning is started, avoid adding extra sugar and salt to home-made foods, and check the ingredients on the baby food tin. Don't overdo the cereal: although this is traditionally the first 'solid' for babies, fruit purees, broth or egg yolk are more nutritious and less fattening. Fresh orange juice diluted with water is better than concentrated juice.

Before putting your baby on a diet, *always* check with the doctor.

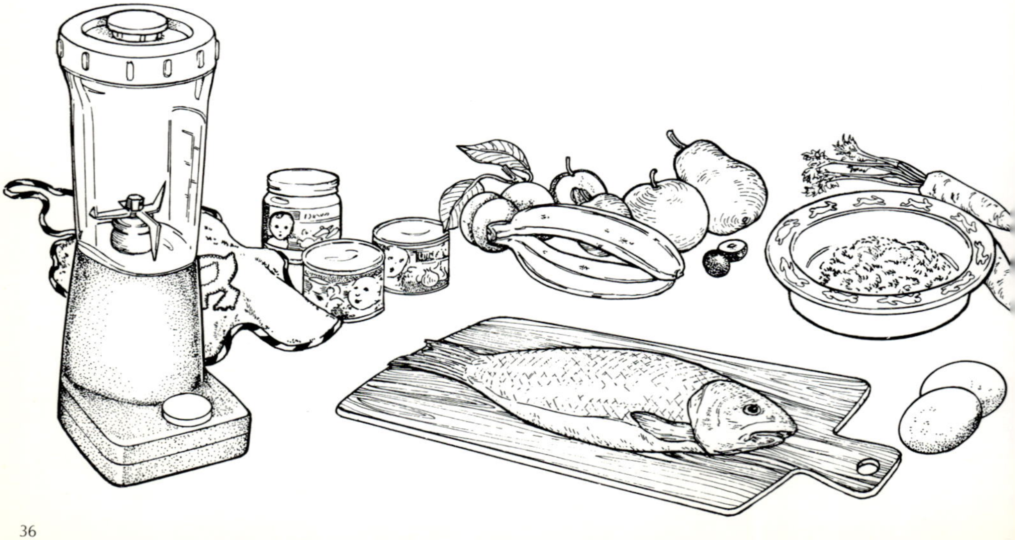

NB These suggestions are a guide only. Check with your clinic or health visitor before putting your baby on any diet.

4 MONTHS
6am: Breast or bottle feed.
10am: Small portion unsweetened fruit puree.
2pm: Home-made broth or strained broth from a can or jar *or* egg yolk; breast or bottle feed; vitamin drops.
6pm: Breast or bottle feed.
10pm: Breast or bottle feed.

Give cooled, boiled water to drink and not sweetened fruit juice (although you could add a little unsweetened juice to the water).

5-8 MONTHS
On waking: Breast or bottle feed.
Breakfast: Apple yogurt (p.58); boiled water with unsweetened fruit juice added.
Lunch: Puree of braised liver in tomato sauce (p.58); egg custard; cooled, boiled water.
6pm: Breast or bottle feed.
10pm: Breast or bottle feed if necessary.

NB At this stage, it's important to make the milk feeds smaller and to gradually drop the last one (maybe you have a sleepy baby who has already dropped it!).

8-12 MONTHS
On waking: Diluted, unsweetened fruit juice or water.
Breakfast: Scrambled egg; wholewheat toast fingers with a little butter; cup of milk.
Mid-morning: Water or unsweetened fruit juice; rusk or piece of apple to chew.
Lunch: Small portion mashed fish or minced meat; mashed carrots; unsweetened yogurt or stewed fruit; water to drink.
Tea: Toasted cheese fingers; small banana; cup of milk.

NB As baby starts to move around, he or she will certainly slim down, but don't rely on this natural process too much: if your baby is frankly fat, then cut out sweet biscuits, cakes, sugary puds and sweet drinks. It's vital at this early stage to give your baby a taste for the *unsweetened* foods!

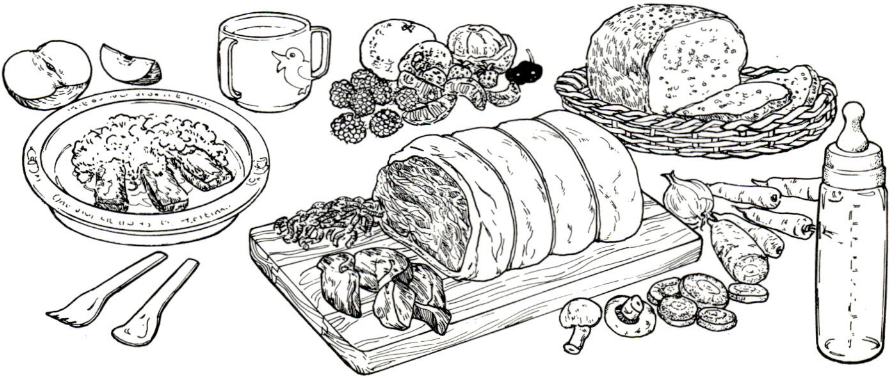

Children's diet

If you've got a fat son or daughter, or even a plump one, *don't* ignore the problem. Fat children often become fat adults.

The only way to help a fat child slim down is to monitor very carefully *exactly* what he or she is eating and to control it as much as possible. School meals are often stodgy, but most schools do now supply salad meals and some allow children to bring packed lunches. Don't give the child pocket money to spend on crisps and sweets after school. *Do* serve up delicious low-Calorie teatime treats which will make him want to come home quickly!

Always serve a nutritious breakfast which includes a protein food for sustained energy, otherwise the child will feel hungry before lunch and possibly visit the tuckshop or snackbar at breaktime. Tuck an apple into his satchel for nibbling on the way home.

Cut Calories subtly by serving grilled foods instead of fry-ups, by using low-Calorie soft drinks, by stocking up with low-Calorie salad dressings, soups and margarine.

About 1500 Calories a day
Daily allowance:
600ml (1 pint) milk; 15g ($\frac{1}{2}$oz) butter.

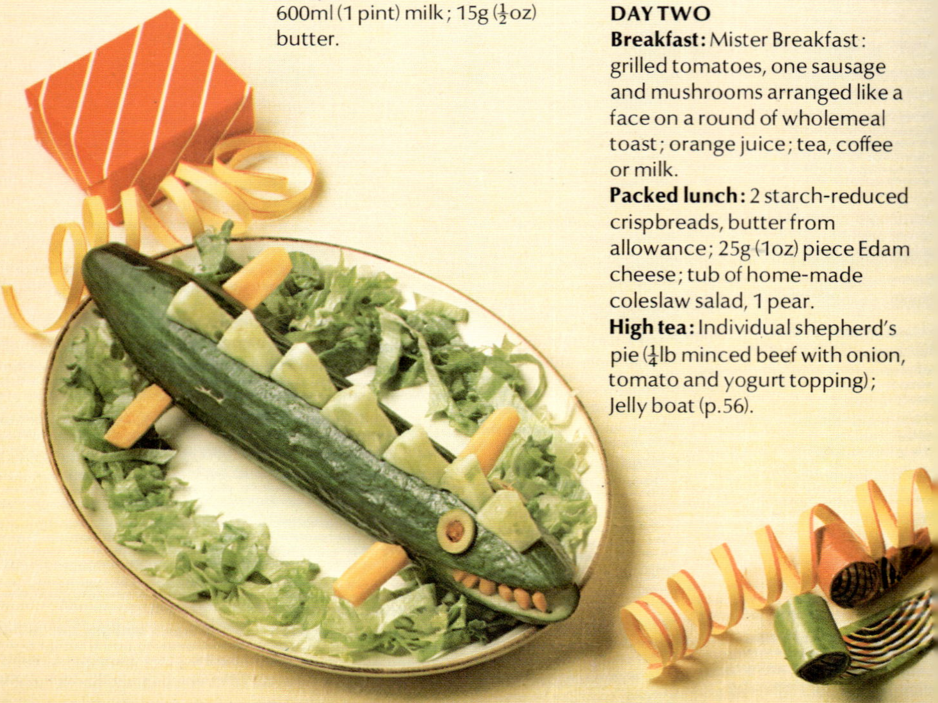

DAY ONE

Breakfast: Egg nest (pile whisked egg white on a slice of wholemeal toast to make a nest shape, slip the yolk in the centre and bake until browned); 1 orange; tea or coffee.

Lunch: Many schools will help overweight youngsters by providing salads and fresh fruit: consult your child's head teacher about this.

Packed lunch: Half a round wholemeal bread sandwich with tuna and watercress; apple; a few raisins and nuts.

High tea: 2 fish fingers topped with grated cheese; grilled tomato; fruit yogurt.

DAY TWO

Breakfast: Mister Breakfast: grilled tomatoes, one sausage and mushrooms arranged like a face on a round of wholemeal toast; orange juice; tea, coffee or milk.

Packed lunch: 2 starch-reduced crispbreads, butter from allowance; 25g (1oz) piece Edam cheese; tub of home-made coleslaw salad, 1 pear.

High tea: Individual shepherd's pie ($\frac{1}{4}$lb minced beef with onion, tomato and yogurt topping); Jelly boat (p.56).

DAY THREE

Breakfast: Small bowl of muesli with chopped banana and natural yogurt on top; tea, coffee or milkshake.
Packed lunch: Small chicken portion with chutney; chopped apple, raisin and nut salad.
High tea: Hamburger face (p.56); mixed salad.

DAY FOUR

Breakfast: Orange juice; scrambled egg on wholemeal toast; tea, coffee or milkshake.
Packed lunch: Cottage cheese tub (use half the cottage cheese and mix with cubes of meat, chopped tomato, cucumber etc., replacing the mixture in the tub and adding a plastic spoon); 1 banana.
High tea: Small grilled plaice with lemon wedge and small portion mashed potato (butter from allowance); plums with artificial sweetener.

DAY FIVE

Breakfast: 2 rashers lean bacon in 1 slice wholemeal bread as sandwich (butter from allowance); grilled or cold tomato; tea, coffee or milkshake.
Packed lunch: Potato parcel: scoop out inside of a baked potato, mix with chopped bacon (grill extra rasher this morning) sweetcorn and seasoning and pile back into skin. Wrap in foil. Pack a plastic spoon. 1 orange.
High tea: Small lean grilled lamb chop; cabbage; apple puree made with artificial sweetener.

DAY SIX

Breakfast: Boiled egg with 'soldiers' of wholemeal toast (butter from allowance) fruit salad; tea, coffee or milkshake.
Lunch: Slice of ham wrapped around home-made coleslaw; separate mixed salad; 1 pear.
High tea: Well-grilled chipolata sausage; cauliflower and carrots; fruit yogurt.

DAY SEVEN

Breakfast: Small bowl muesli topped with chopped apple and a few nuts; milk from allowance; tea, coffee or milkshake.
Sunday lunch: 2 lean slices chicken; peas; cabbage; 1 small potato; frozen mousse.
Tea: Slice of wholemeal toast with 25g (1oz) Edam cheese and tomatoes on top; watercress; milkshake.

If your child qualifies for free school milk the amount consumed at school should be subtracted from the daily allowance.

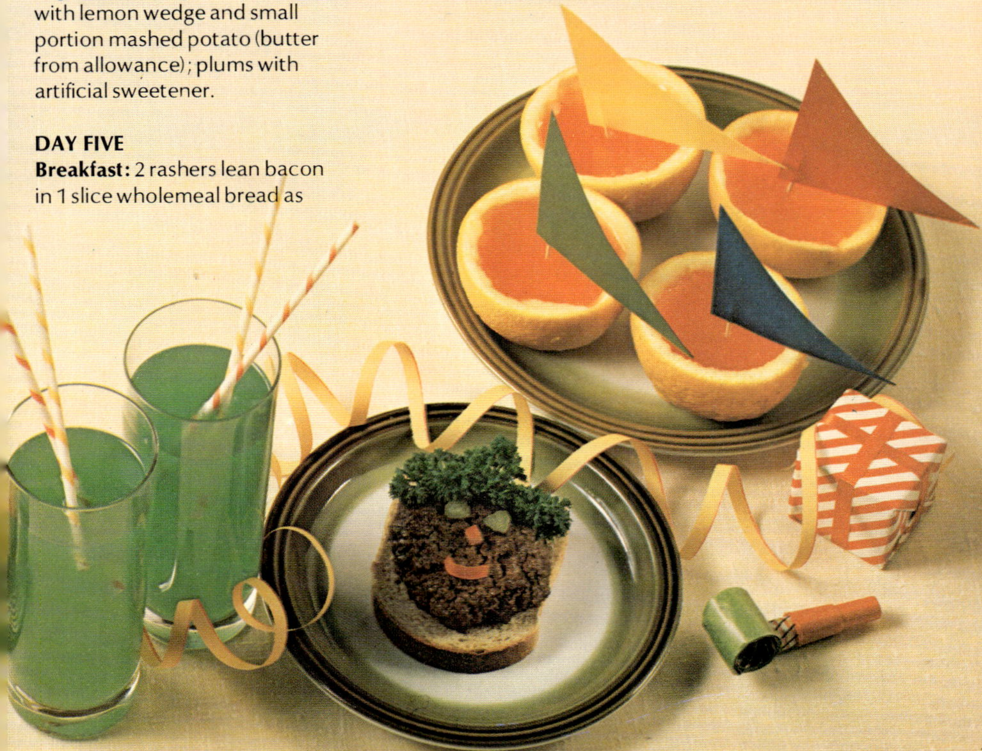

Teenagers' diet

Most teenagers want to look trim, slim, and healthy, and yet this group is most likely to rely on high-Calorie, high-carbohydrate snack foods instead of well-balanced meals as their main source of nourishment. Teenagers who live at home have a better chance of eating well and sticking to a diet like the one below, but those who live away from home frequently find dieting very difficult indeed. A recent survey of teenage homeleavers found that 38 per cent did not eat breakfast, 15 per cent did not eat lunch and over half never ate vegetables apart from potatoes!

The easiest way of planning your slimming campaign if you are a teenager anxious to lose weight is to consider the best possible food sources available to you. If you have to use a school, college, factory or office canteen for lunch make sure you select the most nutritious low-Calorie meals on the menu. If there just aren't any low-Calorie meals available then take your own packed lunch. Start the day with breakfast; if you are in a hurry, whisk up a natural yogurt and an egg with orange juice and nutmeg and *drink* your breakfast. It's as easy to buy fruit as it is to buy a chocolate bar or a pie so get into the habit of buying yourself an apple or pear each day.

If you are stuck in a bed-sitter or college room with limited cooking facilities, stock up on non-perishable foods like low-Calorie tinned soups, starch-reduced crispbread, tinned meats and fish. Eggs are an excellent convenience food and don't need to be stored in a refrigerator. Low-Calorie soft drinks will also help your slimming campaign.

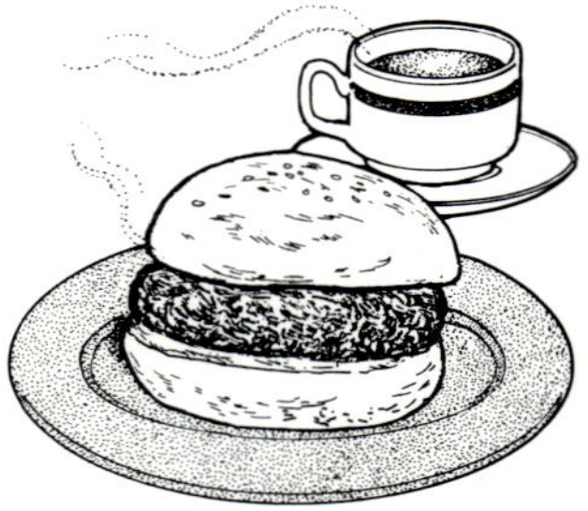

About 1500 Calories

Daily allowance:

275ml ($\frac{1}{2}$ pint) milk; 2 large or 3 small slices bread or up to 6 slices slimmers' bread; 25g (1oz) low-fat spread for spreading on bread and glazing vegetables. Unlimited tea, coffee, water, low-Calorie squash and diet drink.

Now choose one meal from each list plus one snack.

Breakfasts:

★2 boiled or poached eggs
★25g (1oz) any breakfast cereal with milk
★1 carton fruit yogurt
★50g (2oz) thinly sliced or grated cheese toasted on 1 slice bread with spread from allowance
★2 rashers grilled lean bacon or 2 slices lean ham with tomatoes.

Lunches:

★1 grilled beefburger with small can baked beans
★1 beefburger and bun
★50g (2oz) chunk cheese with 2 cream crackers or crispbreads with low-fat spread from allowance; 1 hard-boiled egg; salad
★1 scotch egg with celery and tomato
★75g (3oz) lean ham or corned beef as sandwich (bread from allowance) with lettuce, tomato and cucumber.

Add to all the above 1 piece fresh fruit.

School canteen lunches:

Eat just the main course (no chips!) with fresh fruit to follow.

Evening meals:

★100g (4oz) lean roast meat; 1 medium roast potato; green vegetables; 2 tbs unthickened gravy
★225g (8oz) beef stew or casserole with small boiled potato; green vegetables
★2 grilled sausages with 2 heaped tbs mashed potato; cabbage
★175g (6oz) macaroni cheese with 4 tbs peas
★175g (6oz) grilled or baked white fish with 2 tbs cheese or parsley sauce; small boiled potato and greens

★Curried chicken hot pot (p.59) and Pear meringue (p.59).

Snacks

★1 banana
★2 apples or pears
★1 scoop ice cream
★2 sweet biscuits
★1 tube peppermints or fruit gums
★1 carton natural yogurt
★4 small savoury biscuits.

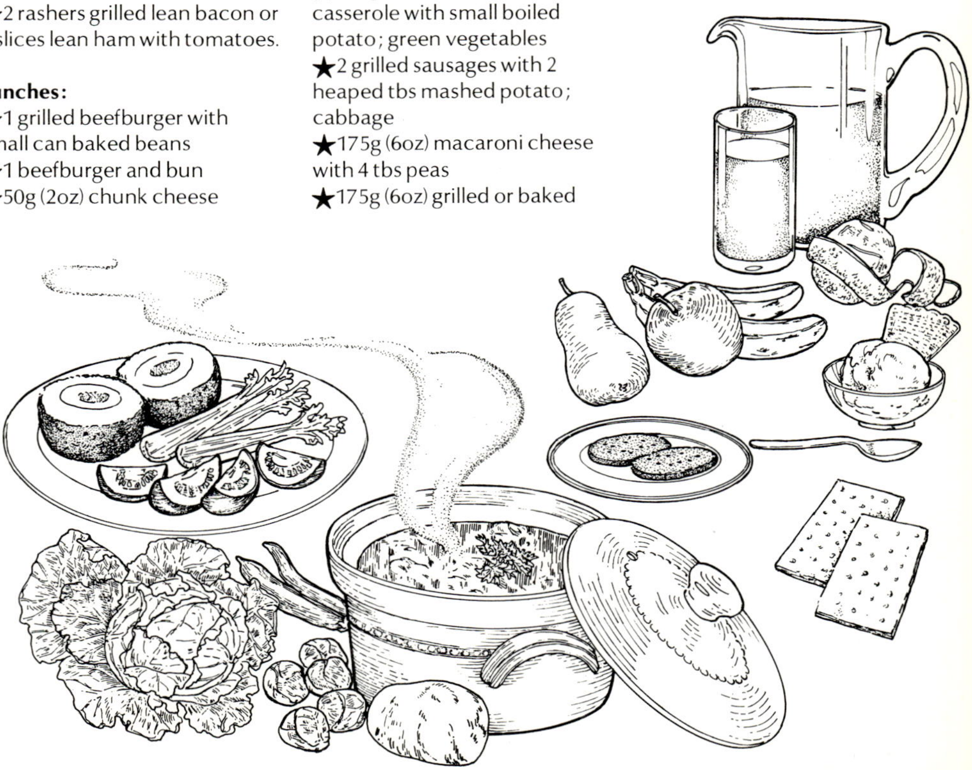

Low salt diet

Many doctors are concerned that the Western diet contains too much salt, particularly 'hidden' salt used in the processing and preserving of foods. Our high-salt diet has been linked with the increase in hypertension and kidney troubles. If you have been advised to follow a low salt diet, try the one below (with your doctor's permission). It will help slim you down as well as reduce your salt intake. It can also be a helpful diet for women who suffer from fluid retention for a week or so before their period and who find slimming particularly difficult and discouraging at that time.

3-day fruit and vegetable fast
Give your body and taste-buds a rest by going on an occasional fast. Weight-loss is often dramatic (although this is usually put back on fairly rapidly afterwards!), and there is a feeling of refreshment and increased vitality at the end of the short fasting period.

However, you *must* make sure that your fast coincides with a long weekend or other restful period: don't cut out vital nutrients when you are working hard or have to be energetic. The diet below should not be followed for more than three days.

About 1000-1200 Calories
Daily allowance:
300ml (½ pint) milk; 12g (½oz) unsalted butter.
Banned foods:
Preserved and canned meats, bacon, tinned and frozen foods, sauces, table salt, dried fruits.

Breakfasts (choose one):
★ 2-egg herb omelette; 1 slice slimmers' bread; small carton yogurt with chopped apple or pear
★ 1 slice slimmers' bread topped with 50g (2oz) cottage cheese and herbs.

Lunches (choose one and serve with large mixed salad with lemon juice and herb dressing):
★ Hard-boiled egg
★ Chicken leg
★ 2 lean slices turkey
★ 50g (2oz) cottage cheese
Add: 1 piece fresh fruit.

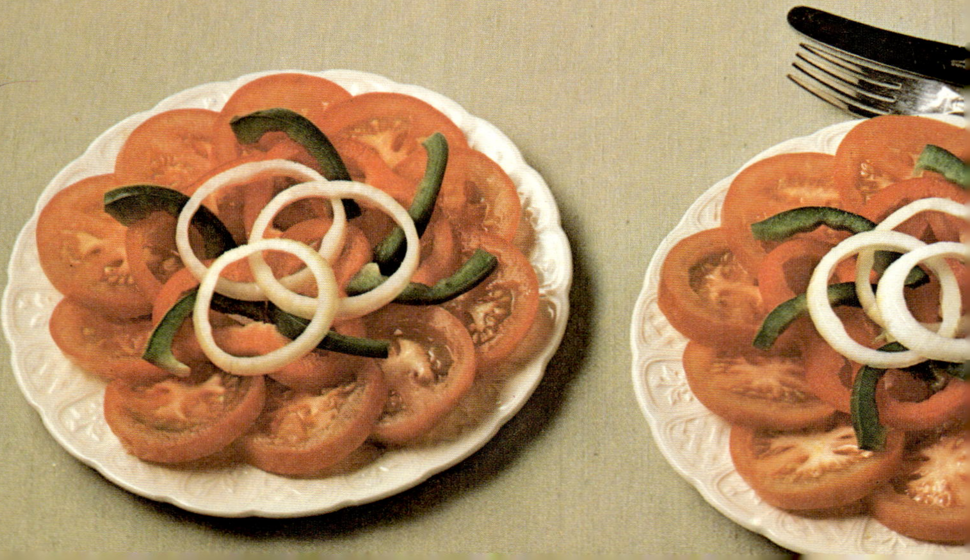

Suppers (choose one):
★Chicken with rosemary (p.57); cabbage and grilled tomatoes
★Lean, fresh meat with large mixed salad with herb and lemon juice dressing
★Green pepper stuffed with mixture of minced beef, onion, fresh tomato, basil, and baked
★2 tomatoes stuffed with unsalted rice and herbs served with cottage cheese and salad.
Hints: Learn to pep-up the flavour of fresh, unsalted foods with lemon juice and home-grown herbs. Read all labels on packages carefully.

3-DAY FRUIT AND VEGETABLE FAST

DAY ONE

Breakfast: Fresh, unsweetened orange juice; chopped apple with nuts and yogurt topping.
Lunch: Orange salad with chopped dates; glass of mixed vegetable juice.
Supper: Avocado and tomato salad; 1 pear and 25g (1oz) hard cheese; glass of carrot juice.

DAY TWO

Breakfast: Fresh, unsweetened grapefruit juice; mixed fruit salad.
Lunch: Mixed vegetables cooked in a little oil with herbs and seasoning; glass of tomato juice.
Supper: Baked apple stuffed with raisins and honey; glass of orange juice.

DAY THREE

Breakfast: Orange and grapefruit segments with yogurt and mint; glass of unsweetened blackcurrant juice.
Lunch: Mixed vegetable salad (use lettuce, tomatoes, celery, cucumber, cabbage etc.) with lemon juice and herb dressing; glass of mixed vegetable juice.
Supper: Boiled cauliflower with tomato sauce; fresh fruit salad; glass of orange juice.

Drinks: Unlimited water or mineral water (the non-fizzy kind).

NB Follow this diet only when you are able to rest frequently, and never for longer than three days. If in doubt, consult your doctor.

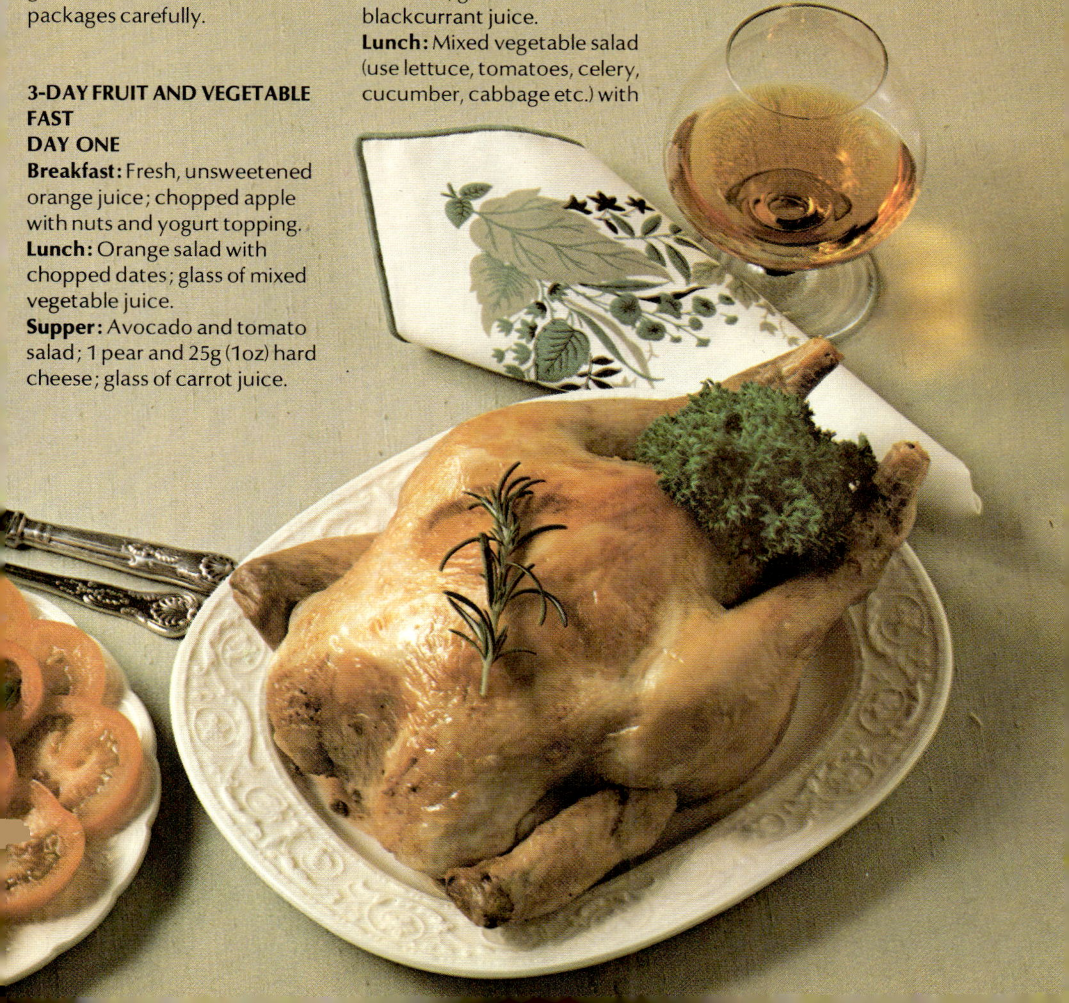

Fitness course 1

The best possible way to shape up while you slim down is to combine your diet campaign with a suitable exercise course. Exercise can help in two important ways: it tones up lazy muscles and helps take up the slack left behind when you lose weight. Regular exercise also helps speed up sluggish metabolism and actually boosts your body's Calorie-burning processes. But to be effective, you must set aside time every day to follow your exercise routine successfully.

The three exercise courses which start on this page have been planned by a physiotherapist to give easy, moderate and fairly tough exercises for the body's top problem areas. Start by following Level 1 exercises and gradually move up the scale when and if you feel you want to tackle something more difficult. In each case you should begin with the lowest number of repeats for each exercise, working up to the highest number in about a week.

Don't rush them: to start with you'll find you need only 10-15 minutes per day. Dress in comfy clothes such as underwear or leotards (jeans are far too restricting for exercising). Select the best time and place for your exercises: you'll need plenty of space. Don't exercise on a full stomach or after a bath. Make sure you are breathing properly: breathe in before any effort and out during the effort. If you start to get short of breath, stop for a few minutes and breathe deeply while lying on the floor to relax yourself.

Keep tabs on your progress by plotting body measurements and weight loss in your diary, or better still on a chart on the wall, but don't expect miracles!

Level 1 These are easy exercises, suitable for most slimmers. However, if you have been ill, have a heart condition, back trouble or other health problem, consult your doctor before tackling the programme.

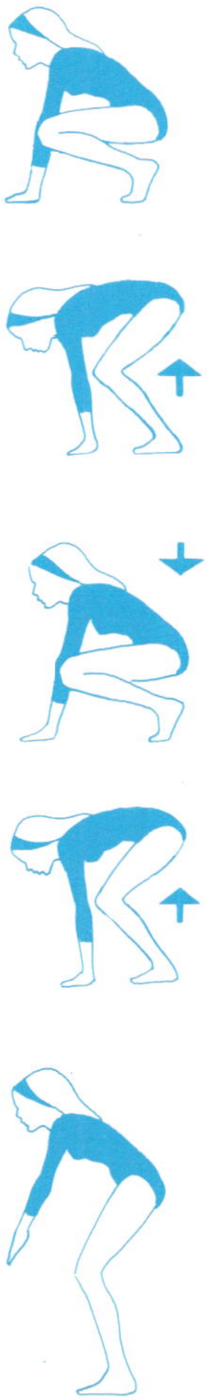

Warm-up: squat, bounce and stretch

Squat down on the floor with your bottom almost resting on your heels and your hands flat on the floor just in front of your feet. Now bounce your knees and bottom up and down twice and then straighten your legs, pushing your bottom into the air and keeping your hands flat on the floor. *Don't* force, just straighten until you feel a stretch in the back of your thighs. Now straighten up your whole body, stretching your arms right up above your head, then swinging them down behind you. Return to the starting position. Repeat 10-20 times.

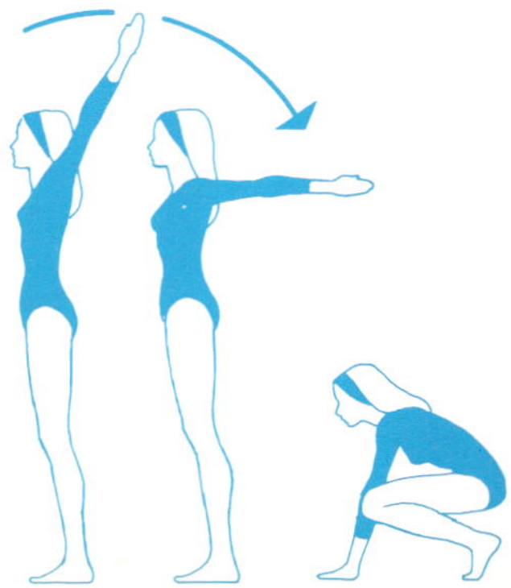

Bust and chest: criss-crosses
Stand with feet apart, raise arms to shoulder height and bend your elbows so that your left fist is level with your right elbow, and vice versa. Now move your elbows in and out so that your fists make fast 'criss-cross' movements in front of your chest. Repeat 15-30 times, remembering to keep your arms at shoulder height.

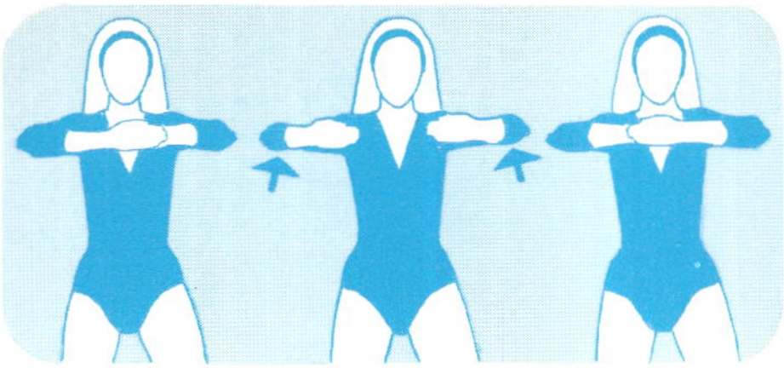

Waist and midriff: side bends
Stand with legs apart, holding a bag of flour or soft canvas handbag behind your head, elbows out to the sides. Now bend your torso from left to right without twisting your body or leaning forwards or backwards. Repeat 10-25 times.

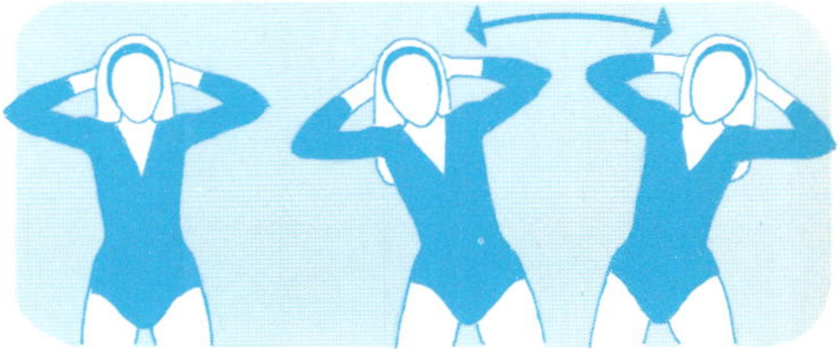

Bottom: backwards leg-raising
Stand at arms' distance from a wall, with palms flat against it. Now raise your right knee to your chest, then stretch the leg downwards and swing it up and backwards as high as you can, keeping it straight. (Don't lean forward.) Repeat with left knee and leg.

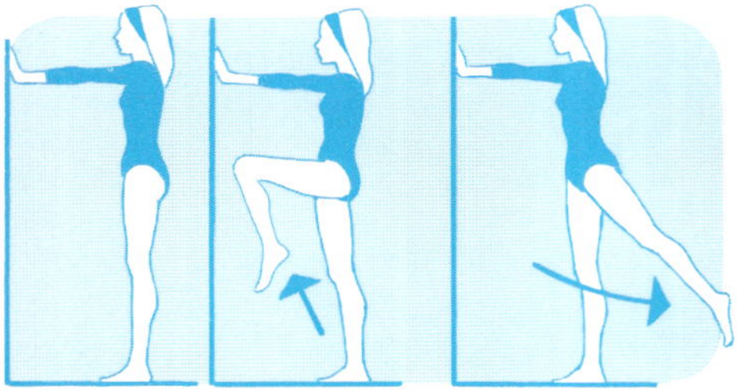

Hips: side rolling
Sit on the floor with left leg straight out in front, right knee bent with your right foot resting against your left knee. Place both hands palms down on the floor behind your bottom. Now roll your right knee over your left leg to touch the floor with the knee without moving your hands. Roll back so your right knee touches the floor on the right. Repeat 10-30 times, then change leg position and repeat with left knee.

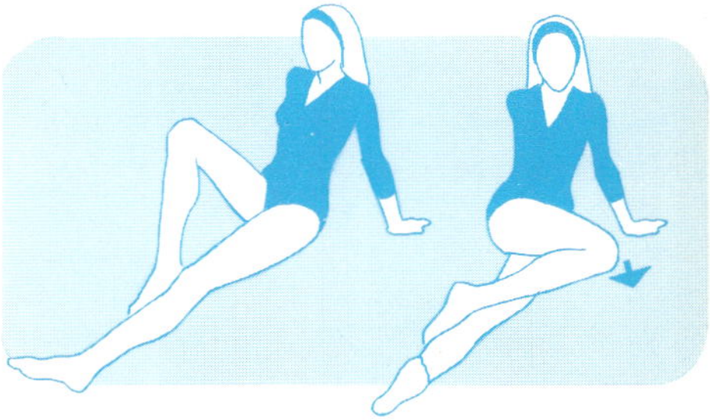

Thighs: split lunges
Stand with both feet on the floor, hands on hips with your right leg straight out in front, left leg straight out behind and legs wide apart. Make sure your weight is evenly distributed between your two feet. Now bend your right leg, moving the weight onto it. Keep your back straight and get as low as you can without leaning forward. Bend and straighten 10-20 times, then swap legs and repeat.

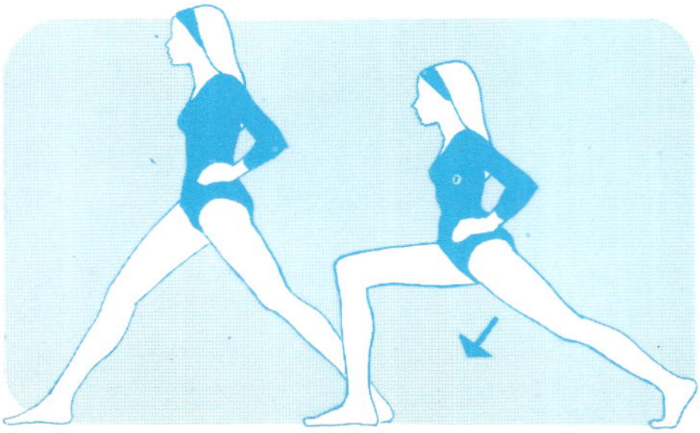

Fitness course 2

Level 2 These are more difficult exercises, but should be fairly easy for the under-20s and those who are older but in good shape.

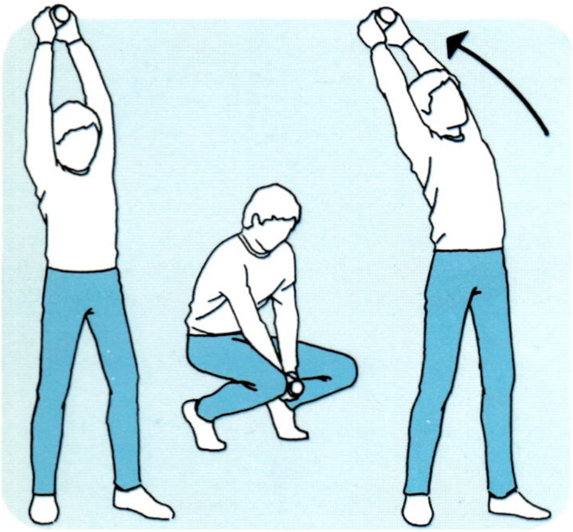

Warm-up: dumbell swings
Stand with your feet apart, clasping a small weight (such as a large can of beans) in both hands above your head with arms stretched up. Now swing your arms forward and down between your legs, bending your knees as you go. Now straighten your legs and swing your arms back up to the stretched-up starting position. Don't forget to breathe in as you stretch and breathe out as you 'curl'. Repeat rhythmically, as fast as you can, 10-25 times. (Left.)

Bust and chest: elbow lifts
Stand with feet apart, hands by your sides, holding two small weights in your hands, e.g. baked bean tins. Bring hands slightly forward. Now raise hands slightly and bend and lift your elbows upwards and backwards, pushing hard. Lower to starting position. Repeat 15-30 times. (Below).

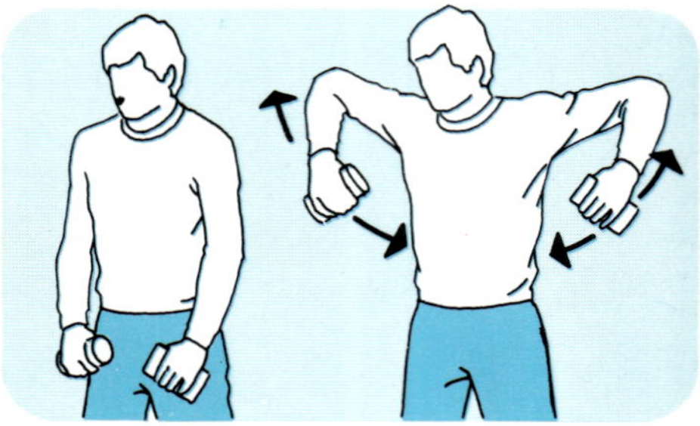

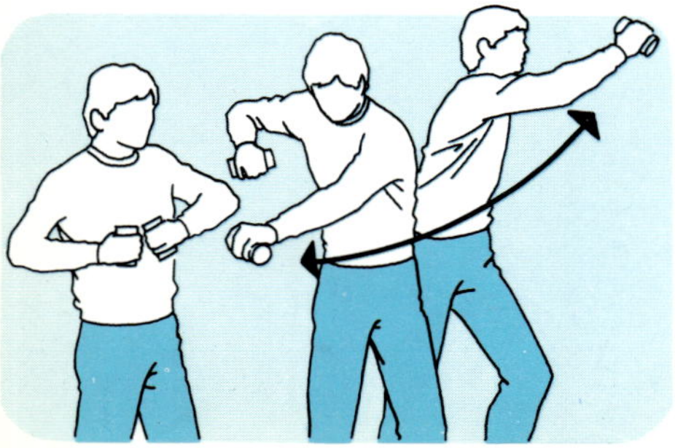

Waist and midriff: twists
Stand with feet apart, holding a weight (e.g. a tin of beans) in each hand. Raise arms and bend elbows at shoulder level. Now punch your right fist hard to the right, twisting round to the right from your waist as far as you can. Return to starting position and punch your right fist to the left, again twisting your body round as far as you can. Repeat 10-25 times.

Stomach: scissors

Lie flat on the floor, hands tucked into the small of your back to support it, with palms flat on the floor. Raise both legs vertically. Now lower your right leg almost to the floor and, as you start to raise it again, lower your left leg almost to the floor so that the two legs cross half way. Repeat this fast scissor action 10-20 times.

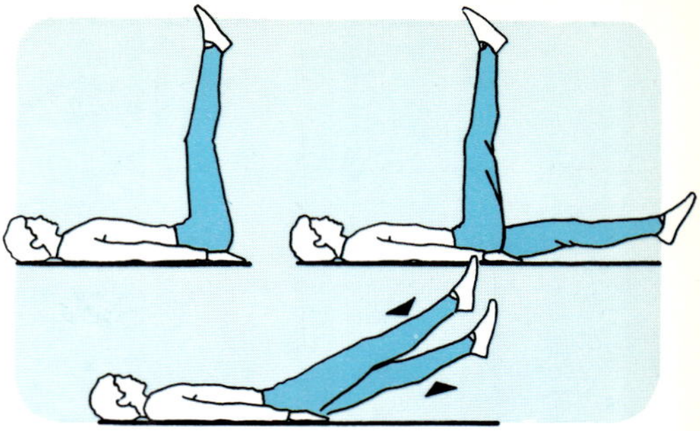

Bottoms: bottoms up

Lie on your back, knees bent, palms and feet flat on the floor. Grip your knees together tightly. Raise your hips and bottom as high as you can and hold the position for a count of five. Now straighten out left leg, keeping it slightly lower than your right knee. Hold for a count of three. Lower leg and body. Repeat whole movement, this time raising right leg. Repeat 10-20 times

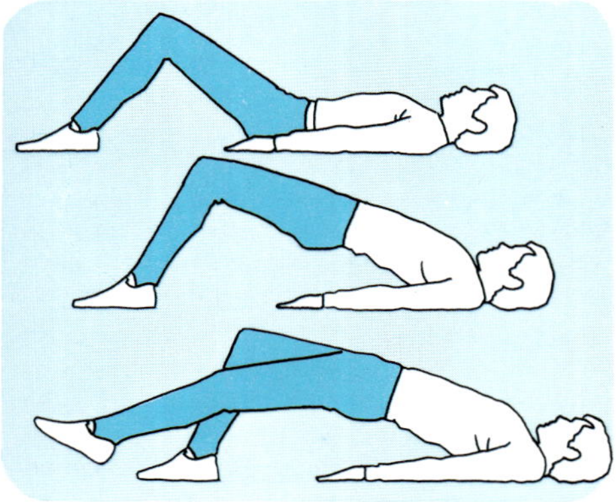

Hips: straight leg crossovers

Lie flat on your back on the floor, arms out horizontally, palms down. Now raise your left leg as high as you can keeping it straight. Flex the foot towards you and cross the leg over to touch the floor on your right as high as you can (you must keep your legs straight and try not to lift your shoulders off the floor). Repeat with right leg 10-20 times.

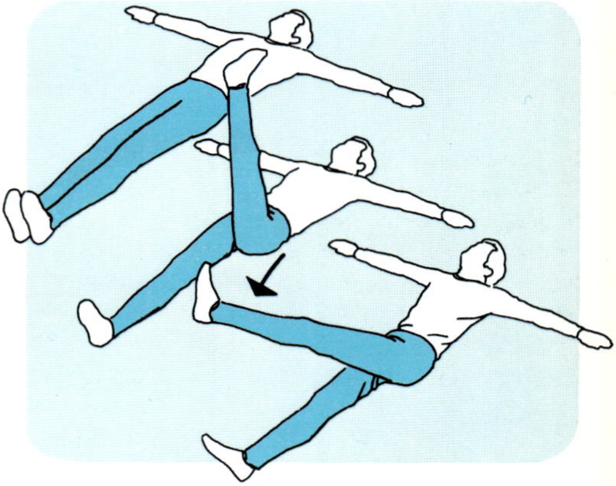

Thighs: split lunge jumps

Stand with hands on hips, right leg forward and knee bent, left leg back with knee bent almost to touch the floor. Now jump into the air, crossing legs so that right leg comes forward, left leg goes back. Allow knees to bend on landing, then jump and cross legs over again. Repeat 10-20 times.

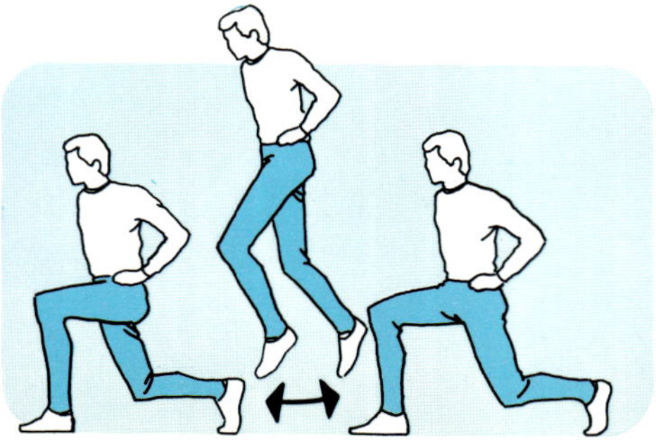

Fitness course 3

Level 3 These are tough exercises and should only be tackled by the really fit. Follow the first two courses for several weeks before attempting them.

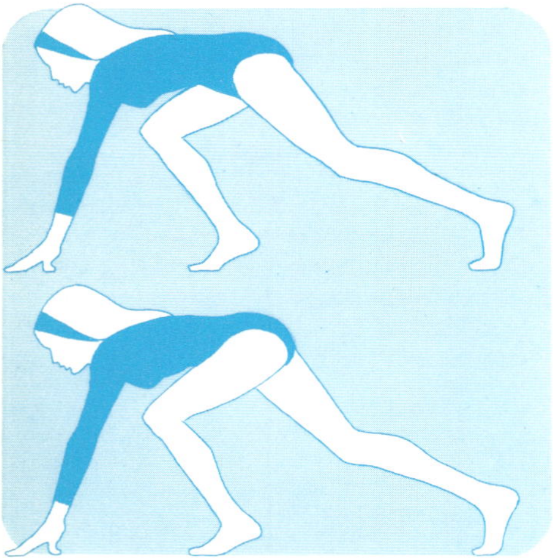

Warm-up: sprints
Squat in a starting block position with the right leg bent, left leg stretched out behind you. Your weight should be on the balls of your feet and hands, which should be flat on the floor just in front of your right foot. Now, with a springing movement, stretch the right leg out straight behind you, and, at the same time, bring your left foot forwards so your left knee is bent. Continue springing your left and right legs out behind you as fast as you can. Repeat 15-20 times with each leg. (Left.)

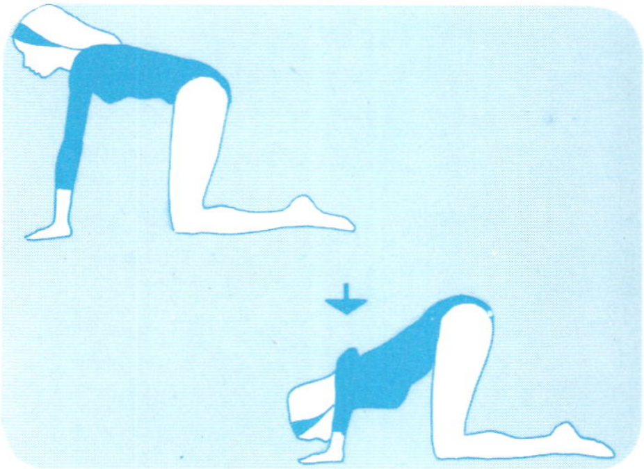

Bust and chest: kneeling push-ups
Kneel down with hands well forward, palms flat on the floor and fingers turned in. Now push your elbows out, lowering your chest almost to touch the floor. Raise up, straightening your elbows. Repeat 10-20 times.

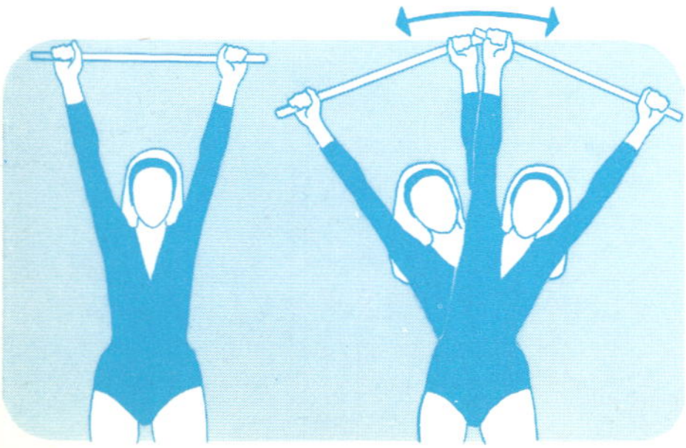

Waist and midriff: oblique sways
Stand with feet apart holding a broom handle or towel with arms straight and hands about a metre apart. Raise arms above your head. Now bend hard to the left, straighten up, and bend to the right without twisting your body or leaning forward. Repeat 10-20 times.

Stomach: knee to chest sit-ups

Sit on the floor with knees bent close to your chest, feet just above floor level and arms straight in front of you with palms down. Now lower legs and body to the floor simultaneously, then return to the original position. Don't arch your back as you lower and raise your body. If necessary, place your hands just behind your bottom to give yourself a lift up and down. Repeat 10-20 times.

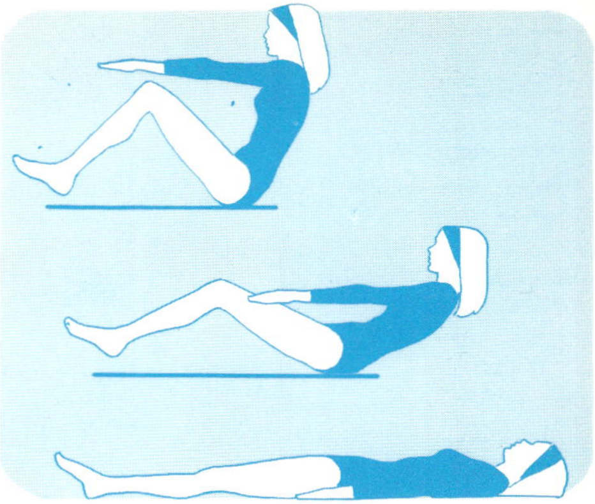

Bottom: thigh lifts

Lie on your stomach, elbows bent and head resting on your arms, legs well apart. Now bend your knees and bring your feet together keeping your knees well apart. Raise your thighs off the floor as high as possible, then straighten your legs and lower them to the floor. You must keep the top half of your body on the floor. Repeat 10-25 times.

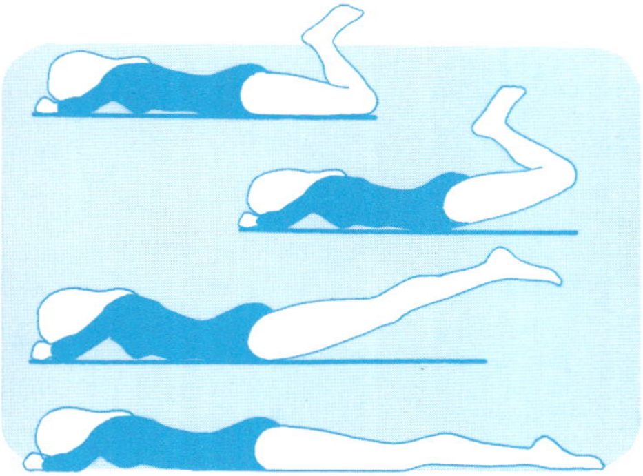

Hips: double leg crossovers

Lie on the floor on your back, arms stretched out horizontally, palms flat on the floor. Raise legs vertically, keeping them straight. Now lower slowly to the right, touching the floor as high as you can. Straighten up again and then lower them to the left. Repeat 10-20 times.

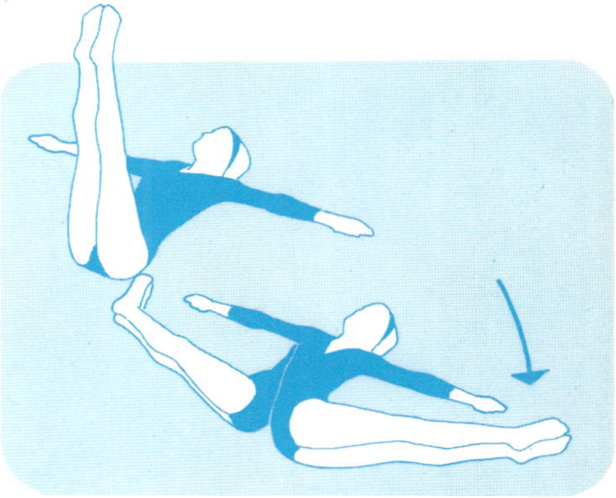

Thighs: backward leaning

Kneel on the floor with knees slightly apart and hands resting on the front of your thighs. Now lean back as far as you can without arching your back. You should keep your arms, back and thighs in a straight line all the time. Repeat 10-20 times.

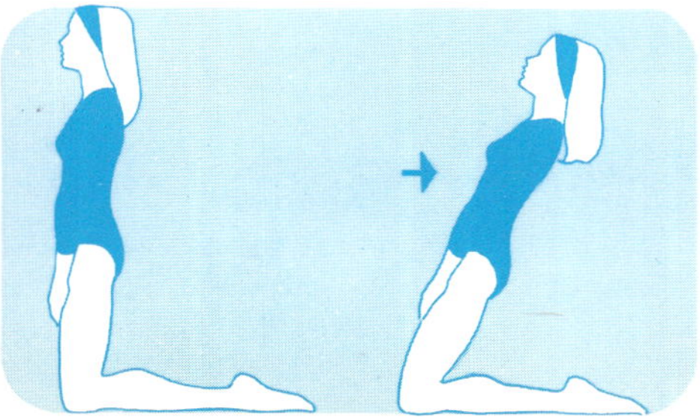

Recipes

On the next eight pages you'll find all the recipes for the special dishes included in the diets on pp. 18-43. Use these with the diets specified or as part of your own Calorie-counted diet plan. Remember that you should aim to cut Calories to 1000-1500 per day.

The recipes include dishes for lunches, high teas, suppers, dinner parties (main courses and desserts), children's parties, teenage gatherings, brunches, and even babies' meals. If the rest of your family are strictly non-slimmers, you'll still be able to find tasty ideas to suit them. Just measure all the ingredients carefully and *don't* add extra fat, sugar, or other high-Calorie items, or you'll ruin the Calorie calculations.

Beef and kidney ring with buttered corn

35g ($1\frac{1}{2}$oz) butter
1 medium onion, peeled and sliced
225g ($\frac{1}{2}$lb) stewing steak
100g (4oz) ox kidney
75g (3oz) breadcrumbs
25g (1oz) wheatgerm
1 level tsp parsley
2 eggs, beaten
150ml ($\frac{1}{4}$ pint) beef stock
seasoning
198g (7oz) can sweetcorn

Melt butter and fry onion, steak and kidney gently for 10 minutes. Remove from saucepan and mince or chop finely all three ingredients; stir in breadcrumbs, wheatgerm and parsley and bind together with beaten egg and stock. Beat thoroughly, season to taste and turn into a 17.5 (7″) greased ring mould. Leave for 30 minutes then bake in a moderate oven (180°C, 350°F, Gas Mark 4) for 45 minutes. Turn out into a warm dish and fill centre with sweetcorn which has been heated and tossed in butter. Serves 4.
340 Calories per portion
1429 kiloJoules per portion

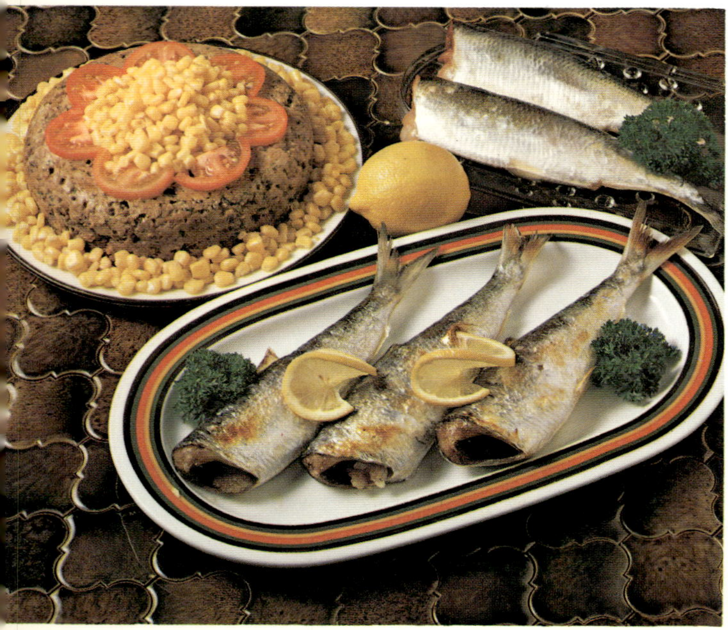

Grilled herrings with mustard butter

4 herrings, 225g (8oz) each
seasoning
flour
25g (1oz) softened butter
1 tsp prepared mustard
1 tsp wheatgerm
squeeze of lemon juice

Remove heads and backbones of fish and clean thoroughly. Sprinkle with seasoning and dust lightly with flour. Cook under medium grill for 10 min-

utes each side. Serve each herring with a walnut of mustard butter, made by creaming all the other ingredients together until smooth. Serves 4.
360 Calories per portion
1512 kiloJoules per portion

Cottage cheese American salad

$\frac{1}{4}$ lettuce
2 fresh peaches or 3 fresh apricots
grapes to garnish
100g (4oz) cottage cheese
50g (2oz) diced ham or luncheon meat
seasoning

Wash and arrange lettuce on plate. Peel peaches or apricots, stone and halve. Halve and pip grapes. Combine cottage cheese with ham or luncheon meat. Season and pile into centres of peaches or apricots and arrange on lettuce. Arrange fruit around it. Serves 1.
360 Calories per portion
1512 kiloJoules per portion

Soufflé omelette

2 eggs, separated
2 tsp water
pinch salt and pepper
1 tomato, sliced
1 tbs chopped parsley and mint
salt and pepper

Beat egg yolks with water, and egg whites separately until stiff. Fold together. Heat non-stick pan, pour in mixture and cook for 1 minute. Top with filling made from rest of ingredients

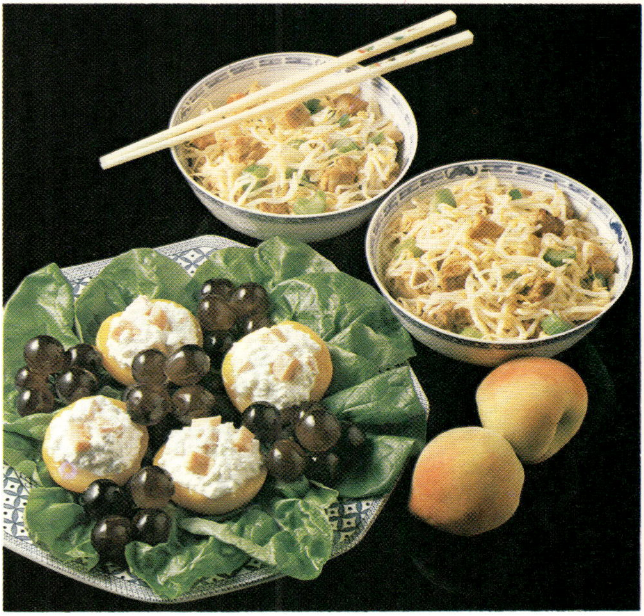

and fold over. Brown under the grill and serve immediately. Serves 1.
170 Calories per portion
714 kiloJoules per portion

Chinese pork with bean sprouts

500g (1lb) lean pork
25g (1oz) butter
1 green pepper
4 sticks celery
1 large onion
150ml ($\frac{1}{4}$ pint) water
1 tbs soy sauce
seasoning to taste
small can bean sprouts

Cube pork and sauté in butter until light brown. Cut pepper into slices, chop celery and onion. Add to pork in pan. Add all other ingredients apart from bean sprouts. Simmer for 15 minutes. Add sprouts and cook for 10 minutes. Serves 4.
300 Calories per portion
1260 kiloJoules per portion

Citrus and avocado salad

1 avocado, stoned and sliced
rind and juice of 1 lemon
2 tbs pure orange juice
2 oranges and grapefruit cut into segments
garnish

Mix orange and lemon juice and brush avocado slices. Arrange avocado with alternate segments of orange and grapefruit on dish. Garnish with cress, orange or lemon peel strips. Serves 4.
100 Calories per portion
420 kiloJoules per portion

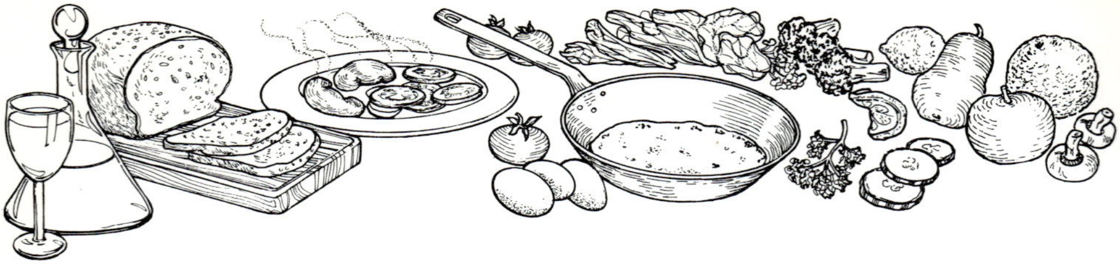

Beef ragout in red wine

1 kg (2lb) skirt steak
1 clove garlic
salt to taste
1 small onion
225gm ($\frac{1}{2}$lb) button mushrooms
2 tbs oil
25g (1oz) flour
300ml ($\frac{1}{2}$ pint) stock
bouquet garni
1 glass red wine
1 tsp tomato puree
chopped parsley

Cut meat into squares. Crush garlic with salt and chop onion finely. Quarter mushrooms. Heat oil in a heavy pan and fry meat quickly until brown on all sides. Turn down heat, remove meat and fry onion until transparent. Add flour and fry for a few moments. Remove from heat and stir in stock, bouquet garni, wine, tomato puree and garlic. Boil. Add the meat and simmer for 2 hours; add mushrooms and cook for a further 5 minutes. Remove meat and reduce liquid slightly. Adjust seasoning and spoon sauce over the meat. Garnish with parsley. Serves 6.
355 Calories per portion
1490 kiloJoules per portion

Veal paprika

1kg (2lbs) pie veal
a little butter
1 tsp paprika
1 small onion
1 clove garlic
100gm (4oz) flour
150ml ($\frac{1}{4}$ pint) red wine
1 heaped tsp tomato puree
150ml ($\frac{1}{4}$ pint) stock
small bunch fresh thyme
or $\frac{1}{2}$ tsp dried thyme
1 bay leaf
675gm ($1\frac{1}{2}$lb) button
mushrooms
lemon juice
seasoning
chopped parsley

Sauté meat in butter until browned. Add paprika, chopped onion and garlic and fry a little longer. Stir in flour. Remove from heat and add the wine, tomato puree, stock and herbs. Simmer for $1\frac{1}{2}$-2 hours. Remove onion and bay leaf. Simmer mushrooms in water and lemon juice. Season and serve mushrooms with veal sprinkled liberally with chopped parsley. Serves 6.
279 Calories per portion
1171 kiloJoules per portion

Fish pie

2 tbs polyunsaturated oil
1 large onion, peeled and
chopped finely
crushed clove garlic
small green pepper, chopped
1 tin tomatoes (large)
1 bay leaf, crumbled
1 tbs chopped parsley
400g (1lb) coley or cod cooked
and flaked
seasoning
110g (4oz) shortcrust
pastry (made with wholemeal
flour and polyunsaturated
margarine)
1 beaten egg

Heat oil and fry onion, garlic and green pepper until soft. Add tinned tomatoes, bay leaf,

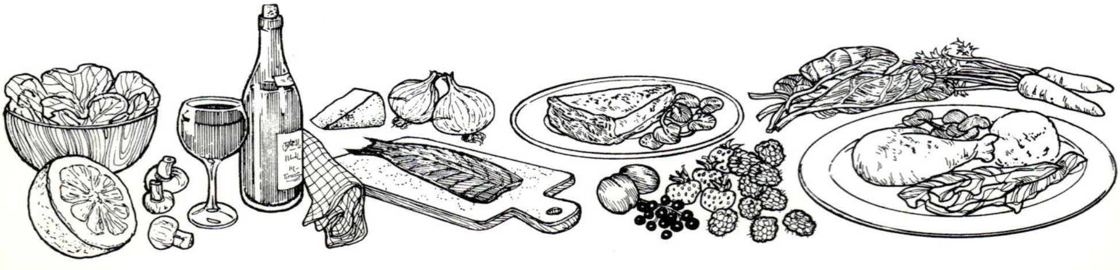

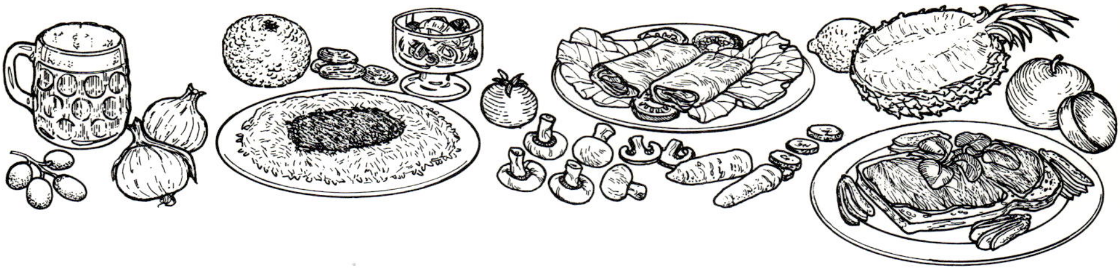

parsley and fish. Simmer for 10 minutes. Season to taste and pour into a 17.5cm (7″) pie dish. Roll out pastry to cover dish and brush with beaten egg. Decorate and make 2 slits for air. Bake at 220°C, 425°F, Gas Mark 7 for 30 minutes or until brown. Serves 4.
335 Calories per portion
1407 kiloJoules per portion

Pineapple crunch

large can pineapple
50g (2oz) fresh wholemeal breadcrumbs from allowance
15g ($\frac{1}{2}$oz) polyunsaturated margarine
25g (1oz) brown sugar
$\frac{1}{2}$ tsp cinnamon
50g (2oz) chopped nuts
small carton natural yogurt

Drain and chop fruit. Toss breadcrumbs in margarine until crisp then add sugar, spice and nuts. Line a pretty dish with the mixture, bake in a moderate oven (180°C, 350°F, Gas Mark 4) for 10 minutes until crisp. Allow to cool, then top with fruit and pour over yogurt. Serves 6.
155 Calories per portion
651 kiloJoules per portion

Vegetable casserole with yogurt topping

15g ($\frac{1}{2}$oz) butter
1 onion, finely chopped
2 sticks celery
100g (4oz) mushrooms
1 aubergine, sliced, salted and drained
2 courgettes
1 level tbs finely chopped parsley
seasoning
Topping:
2 small cartons natural yogurt
3 egg yolks
1 level tsp French mustard

Heat butter in pan and add onion, celery and mushrooms. Cover and cook gently for 10 minutes. Meanwhile, boil aubergine and courgettes in a little salted water until tender but not mushy. Drain and add to pan with onion mixture. Add parsley, season to taste and turn into a 900 ml ($1\frac{1}{2}$ pint) oven-proof dish. Beat together yogurt and egg yolks, add mustard and season. Pour over vegetable mixture and bake at 190°C, 375°F, Gas Mark 5 for 20-25 minutes until topping is set. Serve immediately. Serves 4.
160 Calories per portion
670 kiloJoules per portion

Country soup

4 celery stalks, chopped
1 small turnip, finely chopped
2 onions, peeled and chopped
4 carrots, peeled and thinly sliced
900ml ($1\frac{1}{2}$ pints) vegetable stock (use diluted tomato soup if stock isn't available)
small packet green beans
seasoning

Place all ingredients except beans into a saucepan and bring to the boil. Cover and simmer for 30 minutes. Add beans and simmer for further 10 minutes. Serves 4.
22 Calories per portion
92 kiloJoules per portion

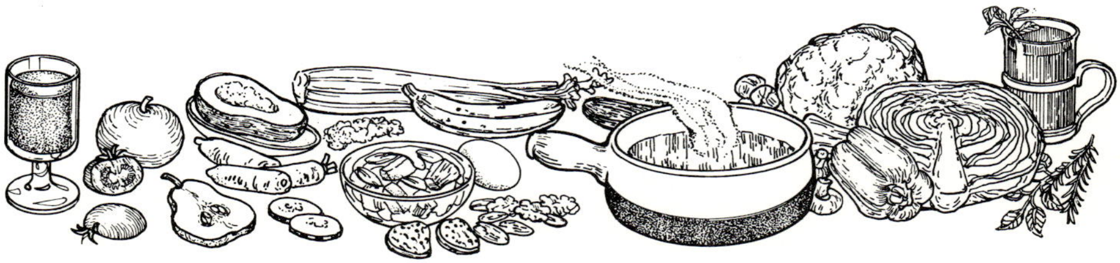

Stuffed lamb

- shoulder of lamb, boned by the butcher
- 2 rashers streaky bacon
- 1 small onion
- 25g (1oz) margarine
- 4 mushrooms, chopped
- 2 sticks celery, chopped
- grated lemon rind
- thyme
- parsley
- seasoning
- sprigs of rosemary

Chop bacon and onion and fry gently in margarine for 5 minutes until transparent. Add mushrooms and celery. Stir in the rest of the stuffing ingredients, and mix well. Use stuffing to stuff bone cavity in lamb, then secure with string. Place in roasting dish with a few sprigs of fresh or dry rosemary and roast in the normal way. Serves 4-6.
440 Calories per portion
1848 kiloJoules per portion

Herring in oatmeal

- 2 small herrings
- 2 tbs medium grade oatmeal
- seasoning
- a little oil
- parsley and lemon wedges to garnish

Clean and fillet fish. Mix oatmeal with seasoning, and toss fish in it. Cook fish gently in heated oil until brown on both sides and cooked through in the middle. Serve with parsley, lemon wedges and Rice and tomato salad. Serves 2.
340 Calories per portion
1428 kiloJoules per portion

Rice and tomato salad

- lemon juice
- seasoning
- 50g (2oz) raw brown rice
- 2 small tomatoes, sliced
- $\frac{1}{2}$ onion, finely chopped
- fresh or dried basil or thyme to garnish

Stir lemon juice and seasoning into cooked and cooled rice. Add sliced tomatoes and onion.

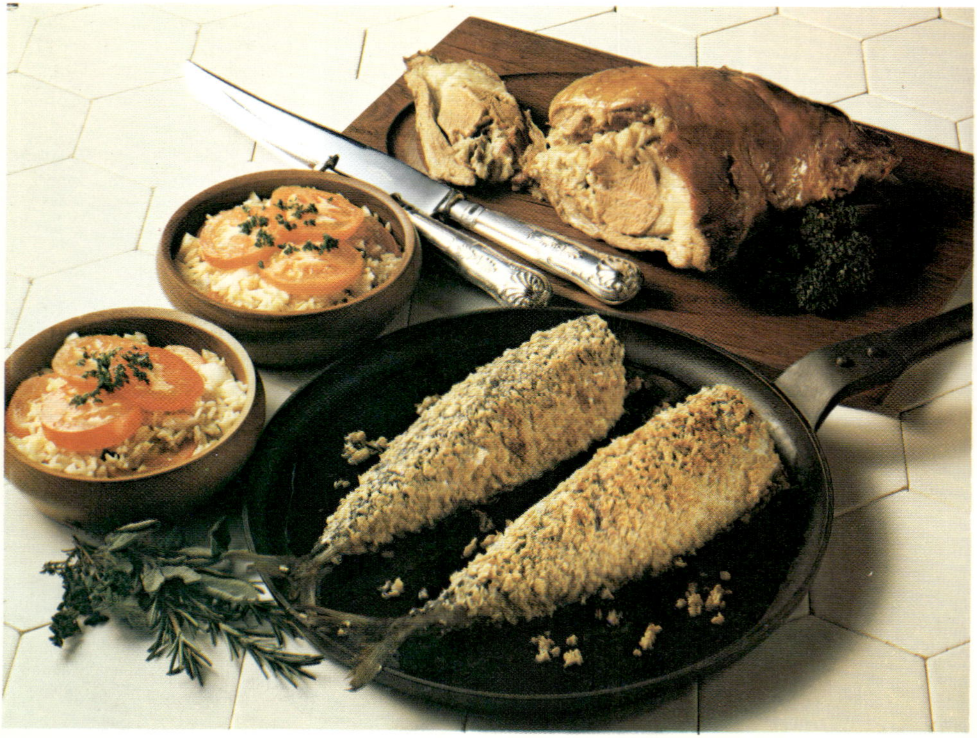

Check seasoning. Sprinkle with herbs and chill for about 1 hour. Serves 2.
97 Calories per portion
407 kiloJoules per portion

Tangy salmon avocado

2 medium avocados
4 tbs natural yogurt
1 tbs lemon juice
1 tsp tomato ketchup
1 175g (7oz) can salmon

Mix yogurt, lemon juice, and ketchup thoroughly. Drain salmon, remove skin and bones and flake fish. Mix salmon into sauce. Split avocados in two, lengthwise, and remove stones. Place on individual plates and divide salmon equally between cavities. Serves 4.
247 Calories per portion
1037 kiloJoules per portion

Dutch peppers

2 green peppers
2 red peppers
25g (1oz) breadcrumbs
2 dessert apples, cored and chopped
3 tomatoes, deseeded and chopped
125g (4oz) Edam cheese, finely grated
175g (6oz) salami, cubed
salt and pepper
½ chicken stock cube
65ml (2½ fl oz) boiling water
1 tsp low fat reconstituted powdered milk
1 tsp cold water
15g (½oz) unsalted butter
15g (½oz) flour
3 tsp French mustard
seasoning

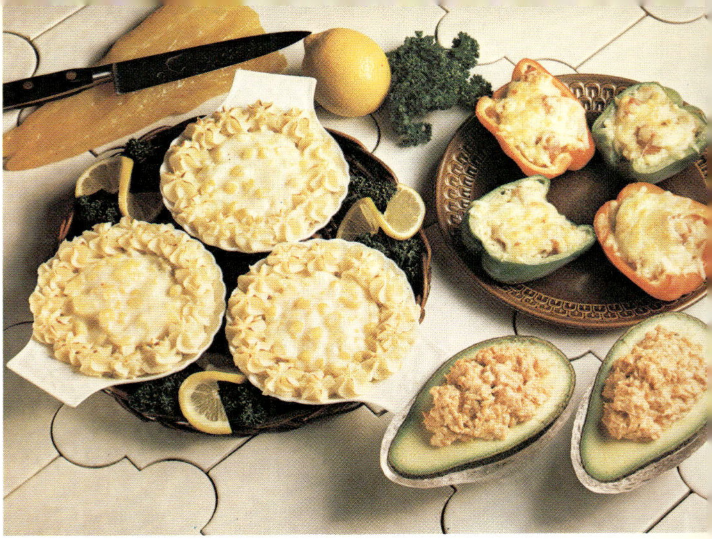

Cut peppers in half lengthways and discard seeds and cores. Blanch in boiling water for 5 minutes, drain and rinse in cold water. Place on oven-proof serving dish. Mix together breadcrumbs, apples, tomatoes, cheese and salami, and season. Make a sauce by mixing stock cube with boiling water, then dissolve powdered milk in cold water. Pour both into a saucepan with butter, flour, mustard and seasoning. Whisk over heat until smooth and thick. Mix sauce and filling and pile into pepper cases. Bake at 190°C, 375°F, Gas Mark 5 for 20 minutes. Remove from oven, sprinkle with cheese, and place under grill until cheese melts. Serves 8.
203 Calories per portion
814 kiloJoules per portion

Haddock scallops

225g (8oz) smoked haddock fillet
150ml (¼ pt) water
25g (1oz) unsalted butter
25g (1oz) flour
150ml (¼ pint) low-fat reconstituted milk
175g (6oz) frozen sweetcorn, cooked and drained
175g (6oz) Edam cheese, finely grated
salt and black pepper
1 tsp each mustard powder and lemon juice
350g (12oz) mashed potato
4 lemon twists
4 sprigs parsley

Poach haddock fillet in water for 7-10 minutes. Drain and flake fish, setting aside water. Make a sauce by whisking together in a saucepan the water, butter, flour, and milk until thick. Stir in fish, sweetcorn, grated cheese and season to taste. Add mustard powder and lemon juice. Spoon mixture into 4 scallop shells or individual dishes and pipe cooked potato around. Grill until golden. Garnish with lemon twists and parsley sprigs. Serves 4.
327 Calories per portion
1308 kiloJoules per portion

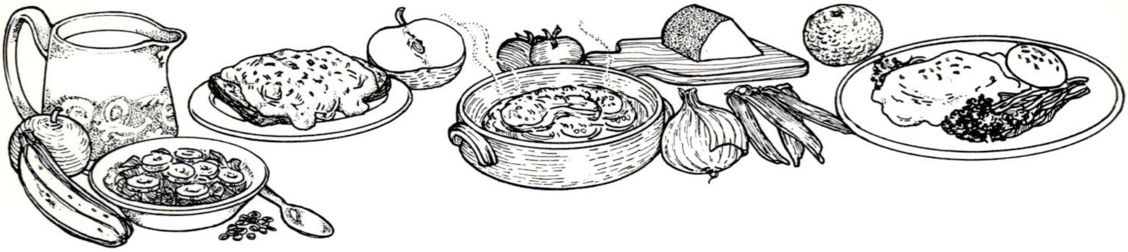

Fish supreme

350g (12oz) any white fish
water to cover fish
2 eggs, hard-boiled and sliced
75g (3oz) Edam cheese, grated
seasoning
2 tbs cornflour
8 tbs skimmed milk
parsley
a few black olives for garnish

Cover fish with the water and poach until cooked. Separate fish from liquid and reserve liquid. Fillet, skin and flake fish, mix with eggs, half the grated cheese and seasonings. Make a white sauce by blending the cornflour with the skimmed milk and 8 tbs fish liquid. Heat well, stirring continuously, until the sauce is thick, then add the fish mixture and cook until hot. Place in an ovenproof dish, sprinkle remaining cheese over the top and melt under a very hot grill. Garnish with parsley and olives. Serves 4.
275 Calories per portion
1155 kiloJoules per portion

Cheese and asparagus flan

Pastry:
40g (1½oz) wholewheat flour
40g (1½oz) plain flour
40g (1½oz) Dutch butter
pinch of salt
water
Filling:
6 asparagus spears, canned or fresh, cooked
2 eggs, beaten
8 tbs low-fat skimmed milk
75g (3oz) Edam cheese, grated
seasoning

Line a 17.5cm (7″) flan ring with pastry made from above ingredients, crimping the edges. Pour the filling made by mixing the eggs, milk, cheese and seasonings into the flan. Arrange the asparagus spears on top in a pinwheel design and bake in a moderate oven (375°C, 190°F, Gas Mark 4) for 30-40 minutes until set. Serve with tomato and onion salad. Serves 4-6.
268 Calories per portion
1126 kiloJoules per portion

Hamburger faces

500g (1lb) minced beef
1 egg
1 tbs tomato ketchup
1 tbs finely chopped onion
¼ tsp Worcestershire sauce
½ tsp salt
pepper
tomato, parsley and gherkin to decorate

Mix ingredients and form into 6 round flat cakes. Grill for 5 minutes, turn and grill other side. Serve on slice of wholemeal bread cut into round shape. Make eyes from rounds of gherkin, mouth and nose from tomato and hair or beard from chopped watercress or parsley. Serves 6.
284 Calories per portion
1193 kiloJoules per portion

Crocodile cucumber

1 large cucumber
1 lettuce
1 small carrot
1 small gherkin
cocktail sticks to secure teeth, etc.

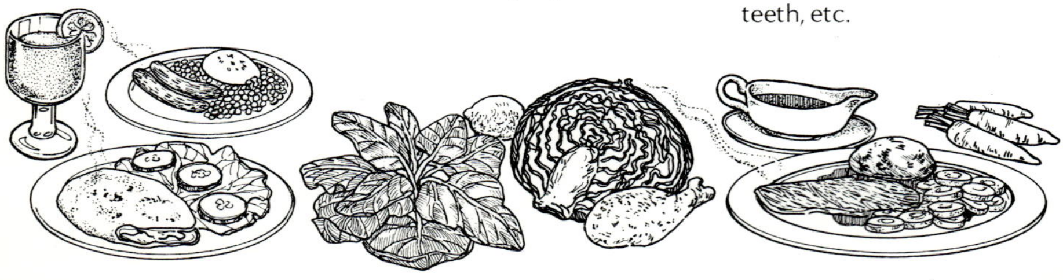

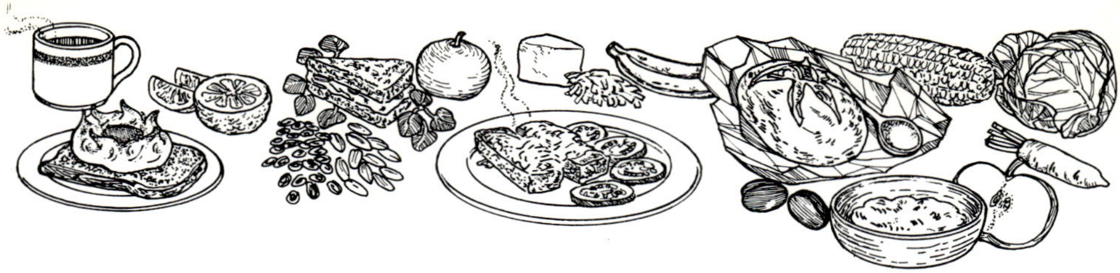

Shred lettuce, wash and drain and arrange on plate. Cut a 'mouth' chunk from one end of the cucumber and insert pieces of carrot as teeth. Insert 4 short pieces of carrot as legs and slices of carrot or gherkin as eyes. For the pointed back of the crocodile, attach triangles of gherkin or a second cucumber. When you've dressed up the cucumber, arrange it on a 'river' of lettuce. This makes a good centrepiece for a party. Serves 6.
11 Calories per portion
46 kiloJoules per portion

Jelly boats

1 orange
1 packet low-Calorie jelly mix
2 cocktail sticks
paper sails

Cut orange in half and scoop out pulp. Make up jelly using orange juice and pulp plus water. Allow to cool slightly, then fill orange halves with jelly. When set, fix paper sails in centre with cocktail sticks. (Write child's name on sail if wanted.) Serves 2.
35 Calories per portion
148 kiloJoules per portion

Lime soda

1 bottle low-Calorie bitter lemon
dash of lime juice
drop of green colouring
ice

Mix and serve on the rocks. Serves 1.
2 Calories per glass
8 kiloJoules per glass

Chicken with rosemary

900g (2lb) roasting chicken
25g (1oz) unsalted butter
1 tbs fresh rosemary, finely chopped
$\frac{1}{2}$ clove garlic, crushed
1 small glass brandy

Heat oven to 180°C, 350°F, Gas Mark 4. Knead butter with rosemary and garlic and stuff inside bird. Roast in moderate oven for $1\frac{1}{4}$-$1\frac{1}{2}$ hours. When cooked, heat a small glass of brandy in a soup ladle, set alight to it and pour over the chicken. When the flames die down, return the chicken to the oven for 5 minutes for the sauce to mature. Served at once garnished with a sprig of rosemary.
300 Calories per portion
1260 kiloJoules per portion

Pepper and tomato salad

$\frac{1}{2}$ medium green pepper
2 tomatoes
1 small onion
juice of $\frac{1}{2}$ lemon
seasoning
parsley as garnish

De-seed and very thinly slice pepper. Skin and slice tomatoes; peel onion and cut into paper-thin rings. Arrange pepper, tomatoes and onion on 4 small plates or 1 larger dish. Moisten with lemon juice, season and garnish with snipped parsley. Serves 4.
11 Calories per portion
46 kiloJoules per portion

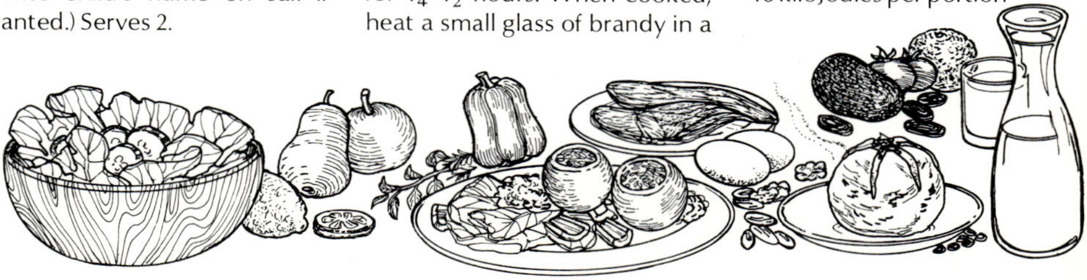

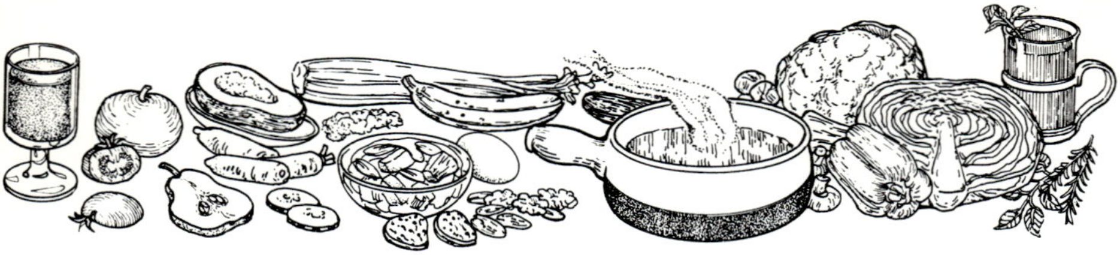

Apple yogurt

100g (4oz) unsweetened apple puree
75ml (3fl oz) natural yogurt
pinch nutmeg

Layer all ingredients into dishes and chill. Serves 2.
40 Calories per portion
168 kiloJoules per portion

Braised liver in tomato sauce

225g (8oz) liver, sliced
1 medium carrot, grated
225g (8oz) can tomatoes
beef stock cube
150ml ($\frac{1}{4}$ pint) water
a little seasoning
chopped herbs

Brown liver slices gently in a pan, then add remaining ingredients. Bring to the boil and simmer for 20 minutes. Puree a portion for the baby, and eat the rest yourself garnished with chopped herbs. Serves 2.
200 Calories per portion
840 kiloJoules per portion

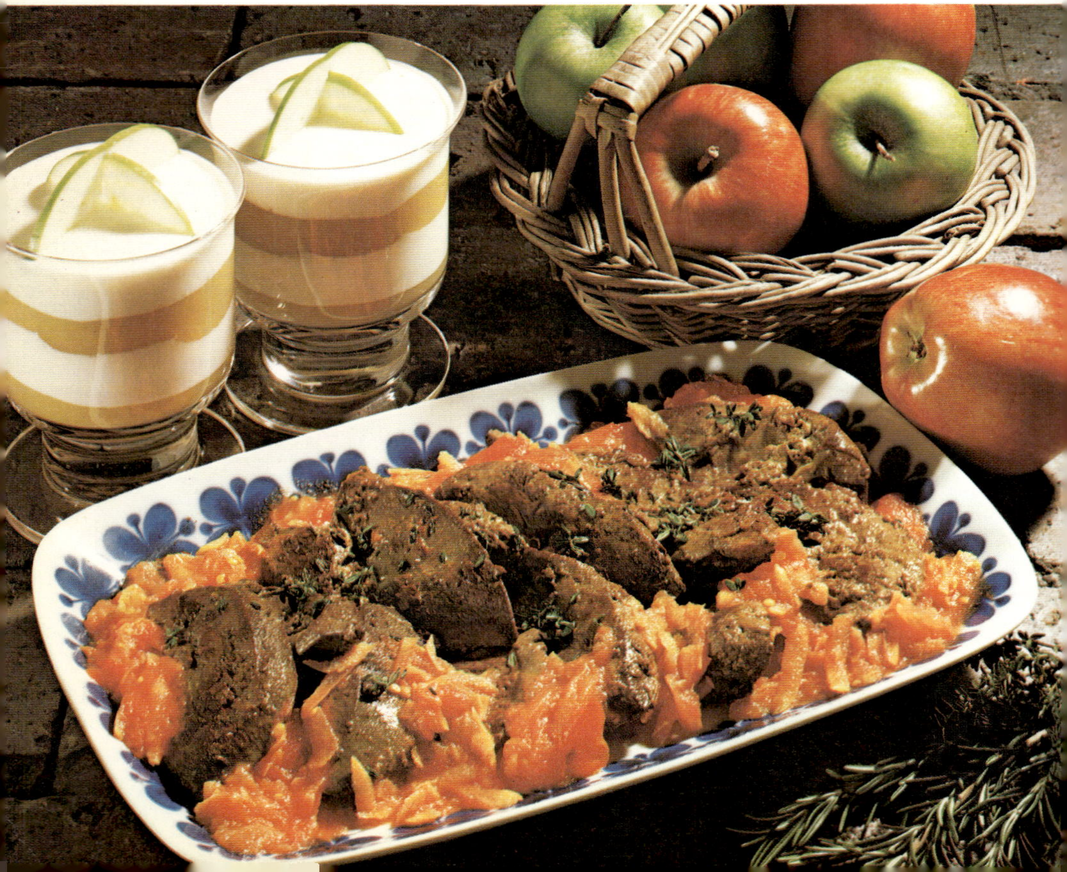

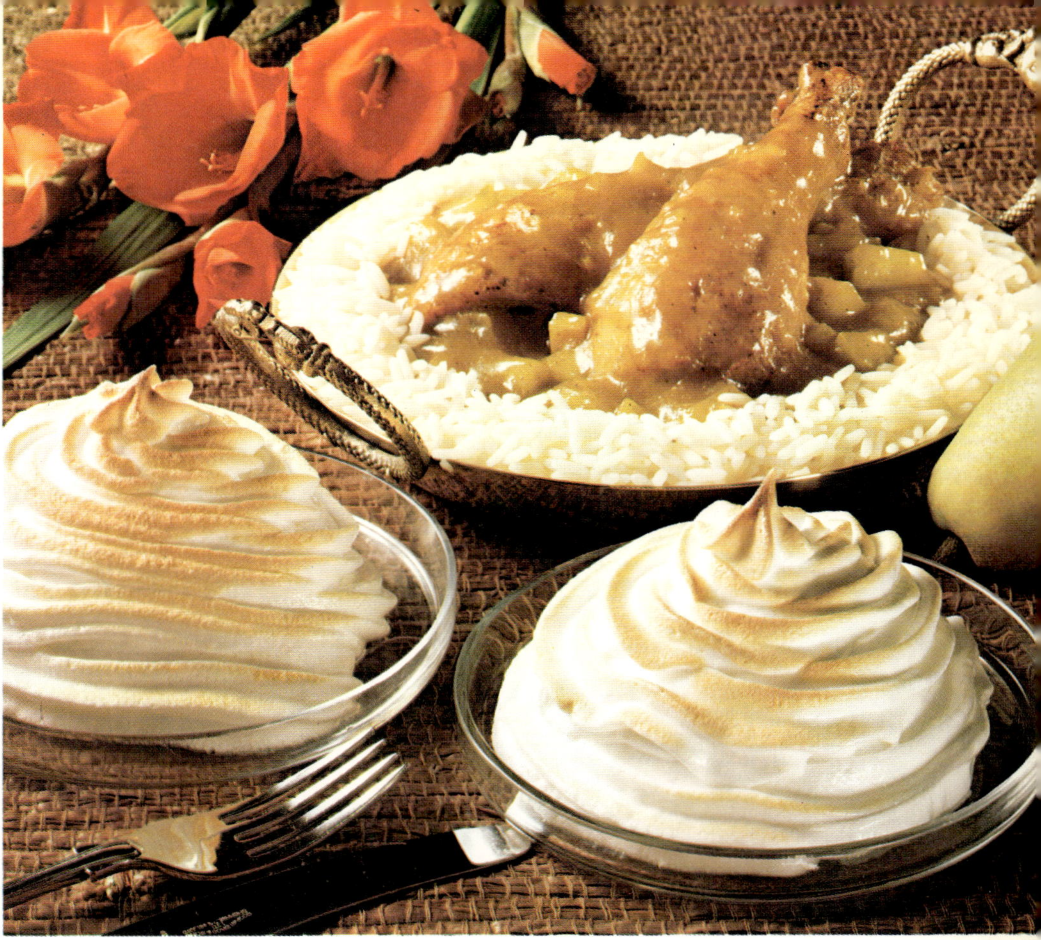

Pear meringue

2 fresh pears
juice of 2 oranges
2 egg whites, stiffly beaten
2 tsp cornflour
liquid sweetener

Peel pears, cut in half and remove cores. Poach in a little water for 15 minutes until almost tender. Drain, place in an ovenproof dish and pour over orange juice. Beat egg white until stiff, fold in cornflour with liquid sweetener to taste. Pile or pipe on top of pears and bake in a slow oven until meringue is set. Serves 2.
70 Calories per portion
294 kiloJoules per portion

Curried chicken hotpot

1 small chicken drumstick
25g (1oz) sliced onion
50g (2oz) diced carrot
1 medium tomato, peeled and chopped
50g (2oz) peeled and chopped apple
300ml ($\frac{1}{2}$ pint) chicken stock
1 level tsp curry powder
salt and pepper
50g (2oz) boiled rice

Place chicken drumstick in a small casserole with vegetables and apple. Bring stock to the boil, stir in curry powder and season to taste. Pour onto casserole, cover and cook in a low oven for about 50 minutes until tender. Serve with rice. Serves 1.
282 Calories
1184 kiloJoules

Calorie, kiloJoule and carbohydrate guide

Use these charts when planning your own slimming diets. Stick to around 1000 Calories (Cals), 4200 kiloJoules (kJ), or 10 carbohydrate units (C.U.) a day (each unit represents 5g carbohydrate), but select the foods which make up a balanced diet as described on p.16.

	Food	Type and size	Cals	kJ	C.U.
Flour-based foods, cereals and pasta	Bread	Slice from large loaf (40g)	105	439	3
		Slice from small loaf (25g)	70	293	$2\frac{1}{2}$
		Slice from wholemeal loaf (25g)	65	272	$2\frac{1}{2}$
	Slimmers' bread	Slice	33	138	1
	Biscuits	2 small plain	125	522	4
		2 small sweet	160	668	$4\frac{1}{2}$
	Breakfast cereals	25g Cornflakes	100	418	4
		25g Branflakes	99	414	4
		25g Muesli	107	447	4
	Crispbread	1 slice, starch-reduced	24	100	$\frac{1}{2}$
	Cake	Medium slice fruit cake	250	1045	6
	Pastry	25g cooked flaky	165	690	$2\frac{1}{2}$
		25g cooked shortcrust	155	648	3
	Rice	1 100g cup, boiled	140	585	7
	Spaghetti	100g, cooked	115	481	5
Dairy food	Milk	600ml fresh, whole	380	1588	$5\frac{1}{2}$
		25g low-fat, skimmed	90	376	$2\frac{1}{2}$
	Yogurt	141g carton, natural	75	313	2
		141g carton, fruit	120	502	5
	Cream	2 tbs, double	130	543	–
		2 tbs, single	60	251	–
	Eggs	1, size 1	118	493	–
		1, size 7	69	288	–
	Butter	25g	225	940	–
	Margarine	25g	225	940	–
	Low-fat spread	25g	100	418	–
	Cheese	Brie, 50g portion	190	794	–
		Camembert, 50g portion	175	731	–
		Cheddar, 50g portion	240	1003	–
		Cottage, 50g portion	60	250	–
		Danish Blue, 50g portion	205	857	–
		Edam, 50g portion	175	731	–
		Parmesan, 15g portion	70	293	–
		Stilton, 50g portion	270	112	–

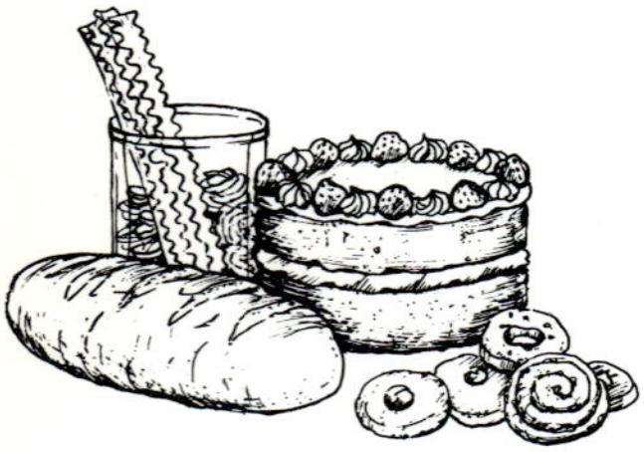

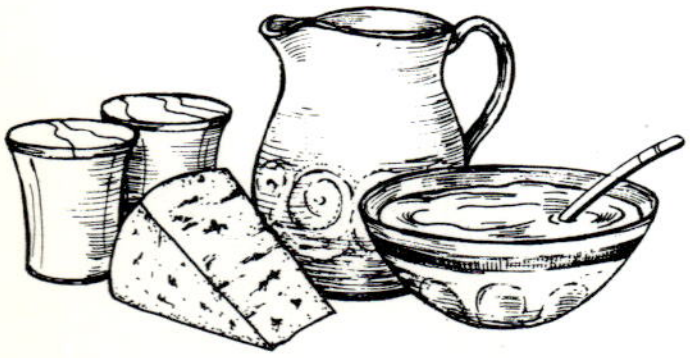

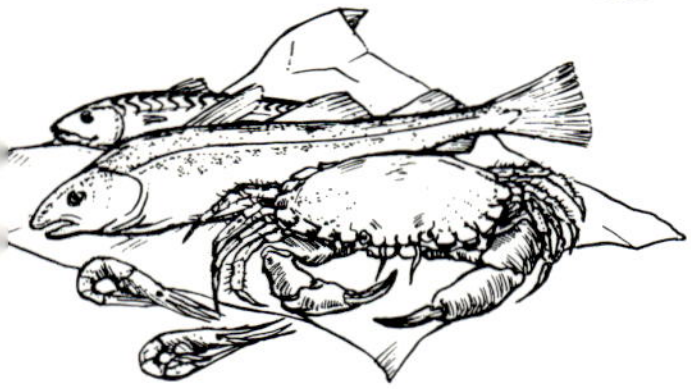

	Food	Type and size	Cals	kJ	C.U.
Fish		100g white fish, cooked without fat	75	313	–
		100g oily fish, (mackerel, kipper) cooked without fat	100	418	–
		175g cod, fried in batter	390	1630	4
		Fish fingers (3)	145	606	$2\frac{1}{2}$
		50g crab	30	125	–
		50g prawns	60	250	–
		Oysters (6)	100	418	–
Meat and poultry	Bacon	2 back rashers, grilled	170	711	–
		2 back rashers, fried	255	1066	–
		2 streaky rashers, grilled	145	606	–
		2 streaky rashers, fried	150	627	–
	Beef	3 slices, corned	130	543	–
		2 slices lean roast sirloin	255	1066	–
		100g grilled lean steak	345	1442	–
		100g stewed steak	230	961	–
	Chicken	2 slices, roast	213	890	–
		265g wing, roast	200	836	–
		90g drumstick, grilled	90	376	–
	Duck	2 slices, roast	355	1484	–
	Ham	2 thin lean slices, boiled	175	731	–
	Kidney	75g, braised	135	564	–
	Lamb	100g chop, grilled	435	1818	–
		2-3 slices leg, roast	330	1379	–
		2-3 slices shoulder, roast	385	1379	–
	Liver	100g, grilled	170	711	–
	Pork	100g chop, grilled	510	2132	–
		2-3 slices leg, roast	360	1505	–
		2-3 slices loin, roast	325	1505	–
	Sausages	2 large grilled beef	310	1296	–
		2 large grilled pork	385	1609	–
	Turkey	2-3 slices, roast	225	940	–
	Veal	100g, stewed	265	1108	–
		100g escalope with egg and breadcrumbs	245	1024	1
Vegetables	Artichokes	100g boiled, globe	15	63	1
	Asparagus	6 spears, boiled	30	126	1
	Aubergine	100g	15	63	1
	Avocado	$\frac{1}{2}$ medium pear	125	522	$\frac{1}{2}$
	Beans	1 tbs runner, boiled	2	8	–
		1 tbs baked	22	91	1
		1 tbs broad, boiled	14	58	$\frac{1}{2}$
		1 tbs butter, boiled	23	96	1
	Beetroot	1 medium, boiled	25	104	1

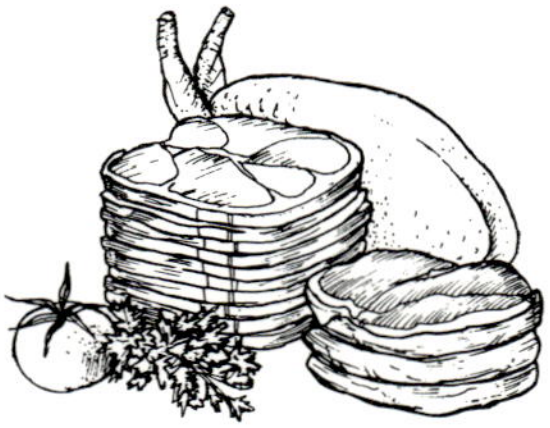

	Food	Type and size	Cals	kJ	C.U.
	Broccoli	100g, boiled	15	63	–
	Brussels sprouts	100g, boiled	20	84	½
	Cabbage	100g, boiled	10	42	–
	Carrots	100g, boiled	25	104	1
	Celery	1 stick	5	21	–
	Chicory	25g, raw	3	12	–
	Cucumber	1 whole medium	50	209	–
	Leeks	100g, boiled	30	125	1
	Lentils	100g, boiled	110	480	4
	Lettuce	1 whole medium	15	63	–
	Marrow	100g, boiled	10	42	–
	Mushrooms	50g, grilled (no fat)	4	17	–
		50g, fried	125	522	0
	Onion	50g, boiled	10	42	–
		50g, fried	200	836	1
	Parsnips	100g, boiled	65	291	3
	Peas	1 tbs, boiled	15	63	1
	Peppers	1 medium, raw	30	125	1
	Potatoes	1 average jacket (200g)	175	731	8
		Medium portion chips	330	1379	8
		1 medium, roast	140	585	5
		Medium portion, mashed	187	782	8
	Radishes	50g	10	42	–
	Spinach	100g, boiled	30	125	–
	Spring greens	100g, boiled	10	42	–
	Sweetcorn	50g, boiled	50	209	2
	Tomatoes	1 average	8	33	–
		50g, fried	40	167	–
		1 tbs, canned	6	25	–
	Turnips	100g, boiled	10	42	½
	Watercress	50g	10	42	–
Nuts	Almonds	50g	340	1421	½
	Brazils	50g	365	1526	½
	Chestnuts	50g	100	418	4
	Peanuts	50g, salted	365	1526	1
	Walnuts	50g	310	1296	½
Fruit	Apple	Large cooking, baked	65	272	3
		Medium, eating	40	167	2
	Apricots	2-3 raw, fresh	30	126	1½
		Stewed, fresh	25	104	1
		100g, canned	40	167	2
	Banana	1 medium	65	272	3½
	Blackberries	100g, raw	30	125	1½
		100g, stewed	25	104	1
	Blackcurrants	100g, raw	30	125	1
		100g, stewed	25	104	1
	Cherries	100g, raw	45	188	2½

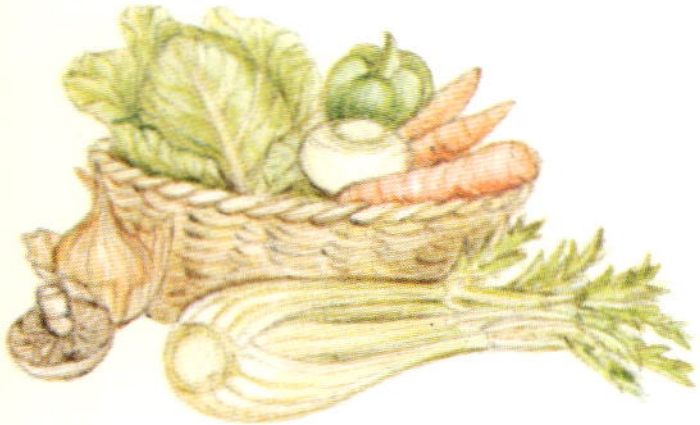

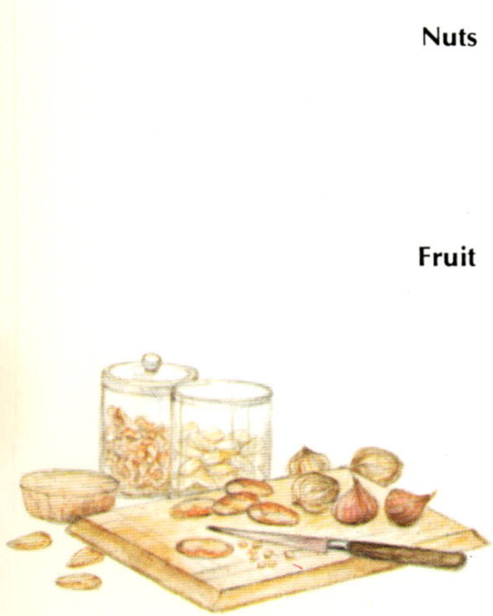

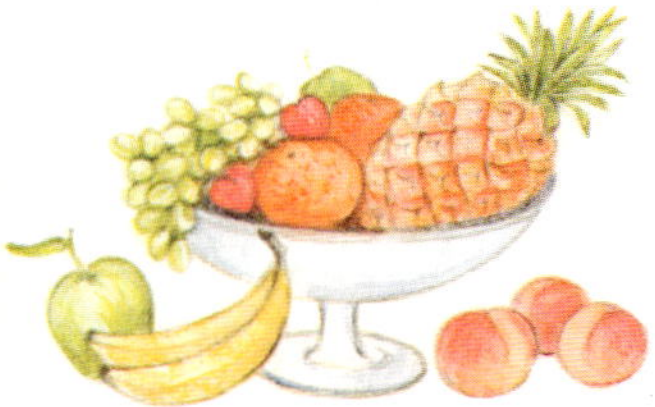

Food	Type and size	Cals	kJ	C.U.
Currants	50g, dried	140	602	7
Dates	about 10	245	1024	12
Figs	3 raw, fresh	50	209	2
	3 raw, dried	245	1024	20
	3 stewed, dried	120	502	6
Gooseberries	100g, stewed	15	62	½
Grapes	100g	70	292	3½
Grapefruit	½ medium	15	62	1½
Lemon	1 medium	15	62	1½
Mandarins	100g, canned	70	292	3½
Melon	1 medium slice	15	62	1
Olives	25g	24	100	0
Oranges	1 medium	40	167	2
Peaches	1 medium	35	146	2
	100g, canned	90	376	5
Pears	1 medium	35	146	2
	100g, canned	90	376	4½
Pineapple	1 medium slice, fresh	25	104	1½
	1 medium slice, canned	45	188	2
Plums	1 dessert	15	62	1
	100g, stewed cooking	25	104	1
Prunes	100g, dried	140	585	7
	100g, stewed	75	313	3½
Raspberries	100g, raw or stewed	30	126	1
Rhubarb	100g, stewed	4	17	–
Strawberries	100g, raw	30	125	1
Tangerines	2 medium	28	117	1

Drink

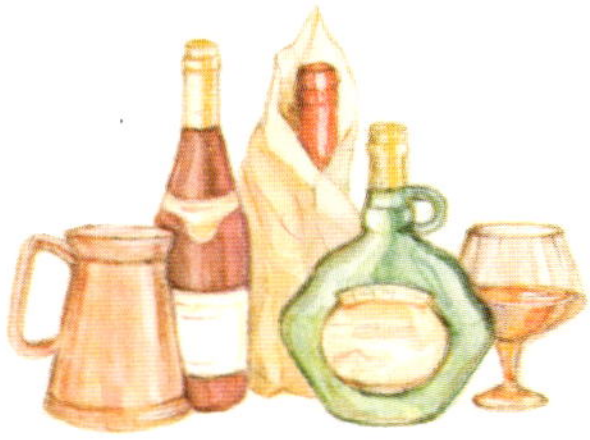

Beer:				
Brown ale	1 pint	160	669	8
Draught bitter	1 pint	180	752	8½
Draught mild	1 pint	140	585	7
Lager	1 pint	150	627	7½
Pale ale	1 pint	180	752	9
Stout, bottled	1 pint	200	836	10½
Brandy	Standard pub measure	75	313	3
Cider	Dry, ½ pint	100	418	5
	Sweet, ½ pint	120	502	6
Gin	Standard pub measure	55	229	2½
Port	Standard pub measure	75	313	3
Shandy	1 can	115	480	5½
Sherry	Dry, standard pub glass	55	229	3
	Sweet, standard pub glass	65	271	3½
Vermouth	1 glass, dry	55	229	3
	1 glass, sweet	75	313	3½
Whisky	Standard pub measure	60	250	3
Wine	Glass, dry	90	376	4
	Glass, sweet	115	480	5

Index

Credits

Consultants
Dr GLS Pawan, DSL London, MRC Path.
Senior lecturer in metabolism, Department of Medicine, Middlesex Hospital Medical School, (University of London) and Consultant nutritionist to the Middlesex Hospital

Exercises on pp. 44-49 were devised by experts at the Westside Health Centre, 201-204 Kensington High Street, W8 6BA.

Artists
John Cameron
Pamela Dowson
Ron Hayward Art Group
Tony Payne
Sid Roderick
Juliette Stanwell-Smith

Photographer
John Lee

Home economist
Carol Bowen

Cover photograph
Peter Myers

Cover design
Camron